T0381372

Love Your Body:

Change the Way You Feel About the Body You Have

Second Edition

Tami Brannon-Quan, Ph.D.
Lisa Licavoli, R.D., C.C.N.

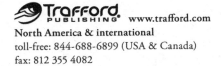

www.trafford.com

North America & international
toll-free: 844-688-6899 (USA & Canada)
fax: 812 355 4082

Contents

Acknowledgments

A special thank you goes out to our clients who we feel privileged to work with on a daily basis. They have shared their stories, struggles and triumphs with us, which inspired us to write the second edition of this book. We have found we truly are a part of a global community. People from around the world send us their stories via our website, www.HealthyBodyImage.com. Our hope is that our book will help all those who struggle with a poor body image.

We are indebted to Stuart Smith and Kathy Li for their editing skills, dedication and belief in our book. Through their meticulous editing the creation of this book was made possible.

Our sincere thanks to all of you,
Tami and Lisa

Forward

&

This book is intended to be used as a guide to help change negative body image. This informative workbook offers concrete, useful tools to assist its readers in exploring and improving body image. *Love Your Body: Change the Way You Feel About the Body You Have* is designed to be an interactive guide. It is full of moving personal stories, case examples, and exercises designed to help readers understand and resolve their food, weight, and body issues; change their negative self-defeating behaviors; improve their "body talk"; practice self-nurturing behavior; and learn to love themselves and accept their bodies. I have known Tami and Lisa for years and their passion for helping women recovering from eating disorders shines through. They began their work in body image transformation many years ago, before it was commonly discussed in treatment. Their pioneering *Love Your Body Workshops* have helped numerous women heal their body image issues. Now with their book they can reach many more people with their powerful message!

Christine Hartline
www.edreferral.com

Introduction

Through our years of experience in seeing clients, we have learned that many women struggle with a negative body image. When asked how they feel about their bodies, most women will respond with a negative comment: "My hips are huge;" "My buttocks sag;" "My breasts are too small," or "I would be so much happier if I could just lose 10 pounds!" These types of negative thoughts and comments are detrimental to a woman's self-esteem and self-image, and they further reinforce the distorted view that, "I am not good enough just the way I am."

There has been a considerable amount of research related to body image dissatisfaction and distortion, especially related to the field of eating disorders. Research done in 1991, found that 81 percent of 10-year-old girls are afraid of being fat (Mellin, McNutt, Hu, Schreiber, Crawford, & Obarzanek, 1991). In a more recent study conducted by Smolak in 1996 it was reported that 80 percent of American women are dissatisfied with their appearance. This same study found that most fashion models are thinner than 98 percent of American women (Smolak, 1996). Another astounding statistic regarding dieting, which was reported in a 1995 study, indicated that 35 percent of "normal dieters" progressed to pathological dieting. Of those, 20-25 percent progressed to partial or full-syndrome eating disorders (Shisslak, Cargo, & Estes, 1995). These statistics are overwhelming, and they illustrate how insidious this problem is and that negative body image issues manifest themselves at a very early age.

As professionals who specialize in the treatment of eating disorders, we have had extensive experience in addressing body image issues. We are dedicated to our work and believe a negative body image is a core issue for many women, not just those women with an eating disorder. A negative body image has a profound impact on a woman's self-esteem and her overall health, and it can literally rob her of the joy life has to offer. We would like to take you on a healing journey—a journey in which you will learn to embrace your body and shower it with love and admiration.

Our compassion and desire to help women heal their body image issues led to the development of the *Love Your Body* Workshop. Together, we designed this workshop solely to address body image issues. The *Love Your Body* Workshop has also been published as a *Facilitator Handbook* (for psychotherapists and dietitians) and a *Participant Workbook*. These books will assist you in making a shift to a positive body image by encouraging you to look inward at all the wonderful qualities you possess as well as to learn to love and nurture the body you have. They are available via our website www.HealthyBodyImage.com.

We designed this book, *Love Your Body: Change the Way You Feel About the Body You Have,* to be an interactive tool to help you heal your body image issues. The more time and energy you put into the exercises and activities we have provided, the more you will get out of the book. It is our hope for you that as you practice the activities in this book you will experience a positive transformation in your body image.

While this book was designed as a helpful tool for creating change, it was not intended to take the place of professional help. If you feel individual therapy and/ or nutrition counseling are needed, we wholeheartedly encourage you to invest in yourself by pursuing these services.

Chapter One

❦

The Growth of Body-Hatred

Many women struggle with negative thoughts about their bodies, and these negative thoughts often lead to profound inner conflicts in their lives. These conflicts can lead to body hatred, which, when taken to its extreme, can lead to the development of fat phobia and eating disorders, including anorexia nervosa, bulimia nervosa, binge-eating disorder, and compulsive over-exercising. For individuals who develop eating disorders, these negative thoughts and beliefs about their bodies become exaggerated, distorted, and obsessive. The body, and all the negativity projected upon it, as well as food and all it represents, become the focal points of the life of a person with an eating disorder—and even the life of many women who do not have full-blown eating problems. The body often becomes the storehouse for anger and negative emotions, thus becoming the "bad" and often hated object.

To address the real issues that are generating the anger and/or other negative emotions, an important shift must be made from an outside focus to an inner one. For many people the thought of addressing their pain squarely in the face is too overwhelming, so they choose to keep themselves focused on the outside— on their bodies, judging its weight, size, and shape.

ATTRIBUTES OF THE FEMALE BODY

The female body comes in a variety of glorious shapes and sizes. General body types include: ectomorph, a very lean build; mesomorph, a muscular build; and endomorph, a rounded build. While we may lean toward one particular body type, most of us are a combination of all body builds. These are God-given structures. We can capitalize on the positives of each type through exercise and diet; however, no matter how much we exercise or restrict our food intake, we cannot shrink our bone size, grow taller, or change our structure.

Most fashion models are thinner than 98 percent of American women (Smolak, 1996).

In today's society, the female body is subjected to unnatural scrutiny and tyranny. If the body is not a particular shape or tone, it's ugly, fat, or unacceptable. If we do not look like 12-year-old boys, does that mean we are ugly? If so, we have lost touch with the feminine principle. Women, as the bearers of children, are designed to have an extra layer of fat to ensure survival of the species in times of famine. Why then do we find it so reprehensible to have a layer of fat? This is a crime—a crime for which countless thousands of women are punished everyday.

It's time we embrace the many wonderful variations of the female form. By honoring the rich diversity expressed through the female body, we come to honor the feminine instead of trying to diet it away. Let's start now to honor the female form in all its variations. Some women have wide hips and some have narrow hips. Shoulders, breasts, and thighs, all come in varying sizes, which makes us unique. As the French say, "vive la différence!" Our goal should be to have an energetic, healthy body that we can achieve with regular body movement and a sensible diet. It is difficult to embrace diversity when the media and society work against you.

CULTURE SHOCK

Our culture plays a significant role in the development of a negative body image. The media, especially television, splashes images of starved models into the viewer's eye, presenting emaciation as feminine beauty. In health spa commercials, for example, the people chosen to act as spa patrons and employees are thin, toned, and often tan. This gives the viewer the message: "If you want to be considered attractive, you need to look like us."

Magazine articles and advertisements also capitalize on the idea of the "fantasy body" by using emaciated models. Many teenage girls and young women look at these women as being representative of the ideal body size and the essence of beauty, a misconception that leads them to try to fit their body size and shape into what they have seen in their favorite magazines. Taken to extremes, this leads to chronic dieting and exercise addiction—the gateway to disordered eating.

The diet industry, a billion-dollar-a-year business, has also perpetuated the myth of the fantasy body. Their message is: "You are not attractive enough until you look a certain way." And their marketing campaigns prey on women with low self-esteem or who have issues with their bodies. These are the women who are most likely to buy their products so they can achieve the "fantasy body." The reality, however, is that the fantasy body is unrealistic for most people—even if they were to take every dietary supplement on the market. In the real world, each individual's DNA determines their body shape and size, and there is nothing they can do about changing it. All they can do is work on making their bodies the healthiest they can be, not changing them into something they were never intended them to be.

The media, especially television, splashes images of starved models into the viewer's eye, presenting emaciation as feminine beauty.

Strive to be the best you can be, not a body type that is impossible.

In the development of body-hatred (See Figure 1.1: *Development of Body-Hatred*), we unconsciously store our worst fears and negative emotions, including shame, guilt, and fear in our bodies. Eventually, we come to believe that our bodies cause these negative emotions. We forget that the body is only the storehouse for these feelings, not the originator.

Figure 1.1: The Development of Body-Hatred

Negative Emotions	Coping Method	Store-house	Transfer of Information	Result
Fear —— Denial —— Body —— Fear of fat —— Body-hatred
Guilt —— Stuffing —— Body —— Guilt for eating —— Body-hatred
Shame —— Displacement —— Body —— Ashamed about how you look —— Body-hatred

In order to fully understand the development of body-hatred we have included the following case study.

CASE STUDY (CARRIE)

As a child, Carrie was told she was fat and lazy. Her parents saw her that way because she would sleep in late on the weekends and did not want to do her chores. What her parents didn't know was that Carrie was a night owl and loved staying up late reading, drawing, or writing. Carrie did not share these activities with her parents because they thought art was a waste of time.

What happened to Carrie through the years was tragic. She came to believe she was lazy, worthless, and yes, fat. Further exacerbating Carrie's negative thoughts about herself was the fact that her habit of staying up late at night coincided with the onset of puberty. During puberty, it is perfectly normal for girls to gain quite a bit of weight as their bodies prepare for the onset of their menstrual cycles. However, no one ever explained this to Carrie. She just assumed her parents were right and adopted their perception of her. The sad part of Carrie's story is that she was actually quite talented and energetic; she just wasn't able to share it with anyone.

Over time, Carrie came to hate her body. She was unable to recognize that she had stuffed all those horrible feelings created in childhood deep inside her body. Instead of recognizing that her negative emotions were a consequence of her everyday life, most notably her childhood, she started believing that her body made her feel bad—her body was negative; she *should* feel ashamed of it; she *should* hate it; she *should* feel guilty about eating.

As Carrie's body-hatred deepened, she developed a poor relationship with food. Her thoughts went something like this: "My body is bad; it's lazy and fat; when I eat I get fat; therefore, eating is bad for me." As a consequence of this thought pattern, Carrie developed a fear of food. She *knew* that if she had just one more bite she would gain weight, which would prove that she was lazy and fat.

Because she had learned at a young age to lock her feelings away, Carrie did not know what to do about the negative feelings that were trying to surface. She could not admit how worthless she felt. The negative feelings stuffed inside her were toxic; the only thing she knew how to do was push them deeper inside her body. This led to more restrictive eating because if she ate, she might get fat, and this would prove to the world that she was fat and lazy.

Carrie became lost in the negative downward spiral of dieting. (See Figure 2.1: *Dieting Downward Spiral*, Chapter 2). Finally, her life became too miserable to handle, and she sought treatment for her eating problems and poor body image.

THE BODY IMAGE AUTOBIOGRAPHY

Loving yourself from the inside out and fully accepting yourself and your body in whatever shape and size God gave you is very freeing and healing. Take the necessary time to reflect, process, and face your fears on the journey to creating a positive body image.

The Body Image Autobiography exercise is designed to identify the progression that led to the development of your poor body image. Take a few minutes to reflect on your own body image, starting with childhood and working your way up to the present day. Think about the first time you remember feeling negative about your body and follow the progression of that negative thought throughout your life. Now write about it. The goal here is to delve as deep as you can into any negative thoughts you have about your body.

How old were you when you shifted from accepting your body to becoming critical of it? This is the place to start your Body Image Autobiography.

_____

_____

_____

_____

_____

_____

_____

_____

_____

_____

_____

_____

_____

_____

_____

_____

_____

_____

_____

_____

_____

_____

_____

_____

_____

_____

By completing the _Body Image Autobiography_ you have become more aware of the progression of your body-hatred. The following assessment is designed to identify how body-hatred is still affecting you today.

THE BODY IMAGE ASSESSMENT

It is important to take a look at your body image and the thoughts and feelings you possess about your body. We have designed *The Body Image Assessment* (See *The Body Image Assessment*, below) a measurement tool for you to use. Before completing *The Body Image Assessment*, make copies for future use. Answer the questions honestly; the assessment is for your information only. After you have worked through all the exercises and activities in this book, you will want to take *The Body Image Assessment* again as a post-test to note the changes that have taken place.

Figure 1.2: The Body Image Assessment

Instructions: For each of the following statements, rate the degree to which it applies to you. Circle only one number for each statement. After rating yourself on all statements, total your points to get your "Body Image" score.

#	Question	Never	Sometimes	Often	Always
Negative Thoughts/Feelings					
1	I feel ashamed of my body in the presence of a special person.	0	1	2	3
2	I feel that other people must think my body is ugly.	0	1	2	3
3	When I walk into a room, I feel the first thing people notice is my weight.	0	1	2	3
4	I feel that friends and family are embarrassed to be seen with me.	0	1	2	3
5	When I feel fat, I have a bad day.	0	1	2	3
	Subtotal				

Negative Self-Perception					
1	I don't like my body.	0	1	2	3
2	I avoid participating in sports or outside exercise because of my appearance.	0	1	2	3
3	I don't like looking at myself in the mirror.	0	1	2	3
4	I don't like to be looked at in public.	0	1	2	3
5	Enjoying activities is difficult because I am self-conscious about my appearance.	0	1	2	3
	Subtotal				

Destructive Behaviors/Patterns					
1	I compare my body to others to see if they are heavier than me.	0	1	2	3
2	Shopping for clothes makes me weight-focused and is therefore unpleasant.	0	1	2	3
3	I am preoccupied with feeling guilty about my weight.	0	1	2	3
4	The number on the scale determines how I feel about myself.	0	1	2	3
	Subtotal				
Now total the number of points you have circled in each column					
					Total Points

SCORING THE BODY IMAGE ASSESSMENT

The purpose of *The Body Image Assessment* is to measure any changes that may occur regarding your body image. If the total points on *The Body Image Assessment* are "0," your body image is exceptional. If the total points are "42," (that is, you circled "3" for every statement), your body image is extremely negative and needs a great deal of work. The basic rule of thumb is: The higher the score on *The Body Image Assessment*, the more negative your body image. *The Body Image Assessment* will give you some indication regarding the level of negativity you have toward your body and an idea of how much work you need to do.

Now that you have completed *The Body Image Assessment*, you have identified areas that need work. It may be in the form of negative thinking or destructive and self-sabotaging behavior. For example, if shopping for clothes makes you more weight focused, do not go clothes shopping when you feel vulnerable. If the number on the scale determines whether you will have a "good" or "bad" day, throw it out. The root of your poor body image issue may reside in your negative thinking. If it seems others are judging your body when you walk into a room, it may be that you are actually judging yourself harshly with critical self-statements. (In Chapter 6, the component of negative thinking in the healing process will be addressed in more depth.)

FIGHTING NEGATIVE THOUGHTS AND DESTRUCTIVE BEHAVIORS

The following activity, the *Toolbox*, is designed to provide you with the resources you will need to combat these negative thoughts and destructive behaviors.

THE TOOLBOX

For change to occur you must think and behave differently. To begin the process of transforming your body image, and to be an active participant in creating change, you will now create your own toolbox for healing.

Use the toolbox as a replacement for self-destructive and negative behavior.

PURPOSE

We want you to treat yourself and your body with love and respect until you can fully embrace the awareness that you are *deserving* of love and respect from yourself and others. As you embrace this realization, treating yourself and your body with love and respect will become more automatic.

SUPPLIES

To build your toolbox, you will need the following:
- A box (no bigger than a shoe box)
- Crayons, markers, or colored pencils
- Pictures, meaningful words or phrases (each word or phrase should have a special meaning for you—and only you)
- Stickers and anything else you feel will help make the toolbox a true representation of you

EXPRESS YOURSELF

After you have gathered all the necessary supplies, start decorating your toolbox.
- Decorate the outside of the box with words, symbols, pictures, and/or images that affirm your body—the external you.
- Decorate the inside of the box with words, symbols, pictures, and/or image that affirm your character—the internal you.

TOOLS OF THE TRADE

Now that you have personalized your toolbox it's time to fill it with the tools you will need to combat any negative thoughts that creep into your head. The tools you place in your box will consist of healthy and nurturing behaviors (e.g., journaling, calling a friend, going for a walk, practicing positive affirmations).
- Cut a piece of paper into 15 small sections (approximately 3in. x 3in.).
- On each piece of paper, write the name of a nurturing activity. Use a separate piece of paper for each activity.
- Place your tools inside your toolbox.

If you choose, you can also share your toolbox with your therapist for any fine-tuning or assistance in adding more tools.

TOOL TIME

Once you have placed all of your tools inside the box, you are ready to begin combating your negative thoughts. This time, however, you will be armed with the tools you need to combat those negative thoughts.

When to use your toolbox:
- When you catch yourself in self-critical and negative thinking.
- When you feel like going on a binge.
- When you feel like eating out of boredom.
- When you feel like eating to push down feelings.
- When you feel like eating and you aren't really hungry.
- When you feel like restricting.
- When you feel like over-exercising.

Anytime you feel overwhelmed or are in a crisis and want to act out with negative behavior, make a commitment to picking out one of the tools from your toolbox. Spend a minimum of 20 minutes engaged in this nurturing activity (the tool from your toolbox). If, at the end of the 20 minutes, the urge is still present, use one of the other tools and do it for 20 minutes. Repeat the process as often as necessary to combat the negative thoughts/feelings or compulsion to engage in destructive behavior.

Ask yourself these following questions:
- Are you really hungry? (bingeing)
- Is food the answer to what you're looking for? (bingeing)
- What real food have you given to your body today as fuel? (restricting)
- Who is in control of you at this moment?
- Who do you want to be in control?

After you have used your tools, take a few minutes to journal (using the space provided below) about the experience and the thoughts and feelings you processed while using your tools. This information will be valuable as you fine-tune what works best for you. The more you practice using your healthy tools the more automatic these behaviors will become when you are feeling overwhelmed and vulnerable to acting out with old, destructive behaviors.

If necessary, feel free to make two toolboxes: one for your home and one to carry with you at work, school, or in the car—anywhere you want to protect yourself from negative thoughts. The toolbox you carry with you can be as simple as a list of all your tools that you keep in your purse.

TOOLBOX EXPERIENCE #1:

_____

_____

_____

_____

TOOLBOX EXPERIENCE #2:

_____

_____

_____

_____

TOOLBOX EXPERIENCE #3:

_____

_____

_____

_____

We commend you for being an active participant in your own healing. You now have the tools necessary to begin healing your body image. Using your tools consistently, on a daily basis, will create your desired change. Do not be surprised when your inner-critic resists the positive changes you are making. Your awareness and diligence in fighting the inner-critic is essential for your success.

Chapter Two

Food Phobia

In our culture, it is nearly impossible not to hate fat—whether the fat is in our food, or on our bodies, or on somebody else's body. We just don't like fat, period. And it is this hatred of fat that leads us to crazy diets and calorie restriction. Rather than following a healthy eating and exercise plan, we too often engage in desperate behaviors, which, when left unchecked, lead to disordered eating. This is because, as several studies have shown, when people restrict the number of calories they consume, their hunger increases. They start obsessing over and dreaming of food. They constantly think and talk about food (Keys, Brozek, Henschel, Mickelsen, & Taylor, 1950), and the longer a person restricts his/her caloric intake, the greater the chance that he/she will overeat later to compensate. This is because when we starve ourselves (whether intentionally or not) we will eat just about anything we can get our hands on, including foods high in fat.

Because we live in a fat-phobic society, and are fat phobic ourselves, we feel compelled to find a way to compensate for those times when we overeat. Some people re-engage in the binge behavior to numb their negative feelings of guilt, shame, and self-loathing. Others turn to some sort of purging behavior. This may be in the form of laxative abuse, over-exercise, or self-induced vomiting. While the purging behavior *may* accomplish what the person set out to do—rid their bodies of unwanted calories—it also creates a great deal of shame.

As this unhealthy cycle continues, shame turns into self-loathing, body-hatred, a poor self-image, low self-esteem, and disordered eating. As we turn our negative feelings inward, we grow to hate our bodies more and more. When hatred of the body reaches critical mass, we develop full-blown eating disorders and food addiction.

People with eating issues hate their bodies. They hate their bodies because the body demands to be fed, and because they feel that the body can never be good enough—it will never look perfect; it refuses to cooperate and be under their total control. Once we accept the concept that fat is hateful, we hate our bodies for even the slightest amount of fat on it. This starts a perpetual downward spiral. (See Figure 2.1, for an illustration of *The Dieting Downward Spiral*.)

Figure 2.1: The Dieting Downward Spiral

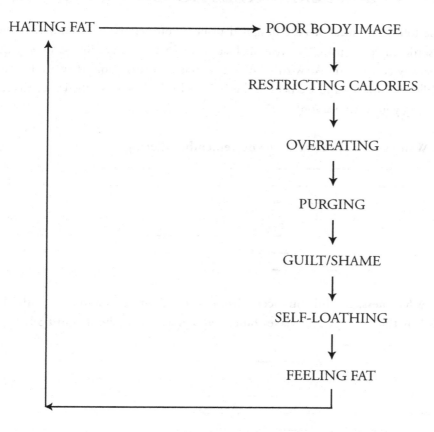

Once a person gets caught up in the web of the *Dieting Downward Spiral*, it is hard to get out of. There is an accumulation of guilt, shame and a complete disruption of normal eating patterns.

A good healthy eating pattern involves eating some fat, occasionally overdoing it, sometimes eating sweets for dessert, or using food in a celebratory fashion. Purging is a dangerous activity and denotes a poor relationship with our body, our food, and our eating. Healthy eating balances intake and output. Purging usually results from days or weeks of limited intake, followed by massive intake: a binge. The shame that stems from purging is often associated with other shameful events in the person's life. Often, bingeing and purging is an unconscious strategy for stuffing hurtful emotions and then ridding one's self of the hurtful emotions through purging. Unfortunately, the shame is perpetuated by the purging behavior.

MY DISORDERED RELATIONSHIP WITH FOOD

The following questions are designed to help you better understand your own disordered relationship with food. Please answer each question as openly and honestly as you can. As with all of the exercises in this book, they are for your edification only—and we believe they will help shed light on the issues that are driving your eating disorder.

1. Write about the first time you remember dieting.

_____

_____

_____

_____

_____

_____

2. What messages did you receive from others about food and your body? Put an * by the messages you have come to accept as truths about your body.

_____

_____

_____

_____

_____

_____

3. What messages did you tell yourself about food and your body? Put an * by the messages you have come to accept as truths about your body.

_____

_____

_____

_____

_____

_____

4. Have the "healthy" and "logical" part of you re-read these statements. If any of them are distorted or false, in any way, change them to a more realistic statement. Use the following as an example.

Disordered Message: *"Chocolate will make me fat. I can't eat it."*

Logical Statement: *"Chocolate on occasion and in moderate amounts will not make me fat. It is not a "bad" food. It's better to let myself have a piece of chocolate than to tell myself it is off limits. When I do this, I set myself up for bingeing on chocolate later. It is this all-or-nothing mentality that fuels my poor relationship with food."*

Disordered Message #1:

_____

_____

_____

_____

Logical Statement #1:

_____

_____

_____

_____

Disordered Message #2:

_____

_____

_____

_____

Logical Statement #2:

_____

_____

_____

_____

Disordered Message #3:

_____

_____

_____

_____

Logical Statement #4:

_____

_____

_____

_____

Disordered Message #5:

_____

_____

_____

_____

Logical Statement #5:

_____

_____

_____

_____

THE PERCEIVED POWER OF FOOD

Part of the healing process in body image work is addressing our food phobias. People who struggle with a poor body image develop a dysfunctional relationship with food and often categorize foods into "good foods," "bad foods," and "in-between foods"—those that are sometimes "good" and at other times "bad." Seeing these words in black and white reminds us just how much power and control we give food. Food is an inanimate object. Innately, it has no power to make you behave or feel a certain way. It cannot make you feel anxious or hateful toward yourself. It is the words you say to yourself about the food and/or eating behaviors that create these negative feelings. And, in order to successfully recovery from your disordered eating, you must desensitize yourself to food and take away the power you have given it.

THE CORRELATION BETWEEN FAT PHOBIA AND POOR BODY IMAGE

As we have discovered, inherent in the hatred of fat is the hatred of the body because the body is where fat is stored. It only makes sense that as the culture came to abhor fat, the culture simultaneously abhors the body, particularly the female body. Fat, food phobia, and negative body image are positively correlated. This is because the logical extension of hating fat is hatred of the body.

THE GREAT FOOD CHALLENGE

To create a positive body image, we must heal our poor relationship with food. The purpose of the following exercise is to make food less threatening, thereby taking away some of its power. There are three parts to this exercise, with space allotted to process and reflect upon your experiences. *(It might be helpful to record yourself reading the following section and replay it later. This will allow you to remain focused on the exercise.)*

Sit comfortably in a chair with both feet on the floor. Close your eyes and begin taking in deep, slow breaths, allowing your body to relax. As you exhale, feel any tension or stress you may have in your body exit through your fingertips and toes. Continue breathing slowly and deeply throughout the guided imagery exercise. Good. Your body is feeling more and more relaxed.

Picture a challenging food…See yourself obtaining this food…Is someone giving it to you?…Are you buying it?…Are you at a restaurant?…Are you driving though a fast food establishment?…

Get the food ready to eat…Remove the food from its wrapper or container… Cook it or reheat it…Whatever you have to do to prepare the food for eating…

Now, see yourself eating this food…Notice what feelings come up for you…

Where are you while you are eating this food?…Are you sitting at a table?… Standing in front of the refrigerator or sink?…Lying on your bed?…Sitting on the floor?…Just take some time to pay attention to where you are as you eat this food…

After you have finished eating, notice how you clean up…Do you hide or throw away your wrappers?…Do you immediately wash your plate?…Do you rinse your mouth out with water or mouthwash?…

Part 1:
Identify a
Challenging Food

Pay attention to all the details surrounding your eating behavior…

Now, take a moment to again focus on your deep and relaxed breathing…

When you feel comfortable, you may open your eyes. You will recall all the necessary details to complete this exercise.

1. Write about this experience from beginning to end.

_____
_____
_____
_____
_____
_____
_____
_____
_____
_____
_____
_____

2. What feelings surfaced for you during this exercise?

_____
_____
_____
_____
_____
_____
_____
_____
_____
_____
_____
_____
_____

3. What were your thoughts in relation to your challenging food?

_____
_____
_____
_____

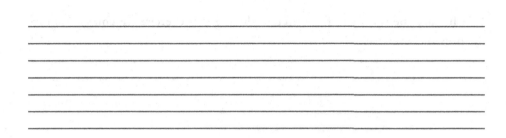

Sit comfortably in your chair with both feet on the floor. Close your eyes and begin taking deep, slow breaths, allowing your body to relax. As you exhale, feel any tension or stress you may have in your body exit through your fingertips and toes. Continue breathing slowly and deeply throughout the guided imagery exercise. Good. Your body is feeling more and more relaxed.

See yourself with this same food…Take in a deep breath, allowing any anxiety or negative emotion about this food to fully release as you exhale…Take in another deep breath and allow all the anxiety and negativity to leave your body as you exhale…

Picture yourself taking away the food's power…This may come in the image of a tug-of-war between you and the food…You may see yourself standing toe-to-toe with this food, like two prizefighters unwilling to concede victory…Or perhaps, you see yourself staring the food down as it circles you like a hungry vulture…Whatever the scenario, see yourself conquering your opponent…revel in your challenging food's demise…

Enjoy your moment in the spotlight…See yourself standing straight and proud, with a sense of inner peace…This food holds no longer holds power over you…You have the power to choose or not to choose this food…You are in control of your eating…

Just sit with this thought and the feelings of peace and serenity it brings… "Tell yourself, I am in control of my eating…"

Now, you can even see yourself enjoying this food—free of all the emotional baggage you used to carry with you…Take in a deep breath and say to yourself, "I am healing my relationship with food!"…"I am healing my relationship with food!"…

Continue enjoying your moment of glory…

When you feel ready, open your eyes. You will remember all the important details of this exercise, and you will allow yourself to continue to experience peace.

*Part II:
Stripping the Food
of its Power*

1. What are the ways you felt different during this exercise (in comparison to the previous exercise)?

_____

_____

_____

_____

_____

2. Did you notice any familiar patterns in your behavior surrounding the food? If so, what were they?

_____

_____

_____

_____

_____

3. Did you notice any shifts in your feelings about your relationship with the food? If yes, what were they?

_____

_____

_____

_____

_____

For the next part of this exercise, you will need a challenging food.

∽

*Part III:
Working with Your
Challenging Food*

Take a few minutes to allow yourself to relax. Sit comfortably with both feet on the floor. With your eyes open, begin focusing on your breathing. Take in a deep, slow breath, allowing your body to relax. Slowly exhale. As you exhale, feel any tension or stress you may have in your body exit through your fingertips and toes. Continue breathing in this fashion throughout the exercise.

Hold your challenging food with both hands. Continue taking in deep, slow breaths while allowing yourself to experience this food. If the food is wrapped, remove the wrapper so you can feel the food…Notice the texture and the sensation of your fingers against the food…

Pay attention to the feelings that are coming up for you. Allow yourself to sit with these feelings for a few moments while you visually focus on and feel the food…Continue breathing slowly and deeply…

Now, take a small bite of this food…Allow yourself to experience the texture of the food on your tongue and in your mouth…Give yourself permission to taste the food…Again, remember to breathe very deeply and slowly, allowing your body to remain very relaxed, as you taste the food…

Good job! You made it through the experiential exercise with the food you have feared for so long. Give yourself a big pat on the back; you deserve it.

Now it's time to write about your experience.

1. Discuss both the physical and emotional experience you had with the food during this exercise.

_____

_____

_____

_____

_____

_____

_____

_____

_____

_____

_____

2. Fill in the blank: "This food makes me feel":

_____

_____

_____

3. Rephrase the above statement with an "I" statement (e.g., "I feel anxious when I see a brownie.").

_____

_____

_____

4. Write about the power you give to this inanimate object called food.

_____

_____

_____

_____

☙

Challenge
The next time you find yourself saying, "This food makes me feel….", replace it with an "I" statement. Explore the reality that you do have a choice about the way you feel.

_____
_____
_____
_____
_____

The Creation of an Eating Disorder

The creation of an eating disorder/disordered eating is multifactorial. Fat phobia and poor body image help to create, and are significant characteristics of, an eating disorder/disordered eating. There is also extreme societal pressure for women to look a certain way, which creates disordered eating and, in its extreme form, an eating disorder.

ℋ

Learning to love and respect your body is essential for healing.

Age is not the determining factor in whether an individual develops disordered eating or an eating disordered. In fact, we are seeing a very broad spectrum in age from prepubescent females at nine years old to women in their 40s and 50s struggling with body image issues that result in disordered eating and can lead to the development of full-blown eating disorders. In recent years, we have seen a growth in the plastic surgery and anti-aging industries. This has put even more pressure on women to achieve a "perfect" body. Middle-aged women are very vulnerable to developing disordered eating as their body's age. If a woman has not developed her inner self, then the wrinkling, sagging, and graying hair, all of which are natural parts of the aging process, may put her into a tailspin.

There are certain factors that make some more susceptible to developing an eating disorder/disordered eating. This includes being raised in an environment in which there is abuse (emotional, physical, or sexual) or criticism. Additional factors include dysfunctional families or desiring perfection (a goal, which, as human beings, is unattainable). When coupled with social pressures or the expectations the media places on women, any one of these factors can easily lead to the development of an eating disorder/disordered eating.

Figure 2.2: *The Creation of an Eating Disorder/Disordered Eating* gives a visual representation of just how an eating disorder/disordered eating is created.

Figure 2.2: The Creation of an Eating Disorder/Disordered Eating

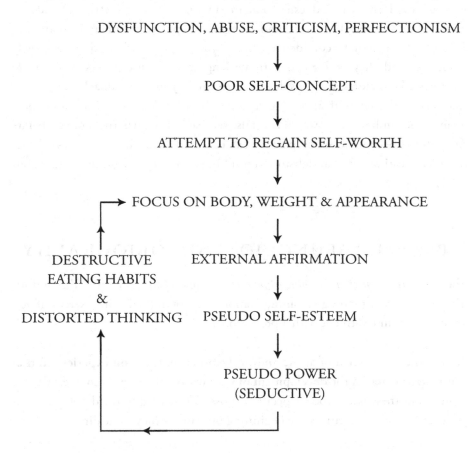

DYSFUNCTION, ABUSE, CRITICISM, PERFECTIONISM

↓

POOR SELF-CONCEPT

↓

ATTEMPT TO REGAIN SELF-WORTH

↓

FOCUS ON BODY, WEIGHT & APPEARANCE

↓

EXTERNAL AFFIRMATION

↓

PSEUDO SELF-ESTEEM

↓

PSEUDO POWER
(SEDUCTIVE)

DESTRUCTIVE
EATING HABITS
&
DISTORTED THINKING

In the diagram, we see that early childhood dysfunction, abuse, criticism, and perfectionism can lead to the development of an eating disorder/disordered eating. Children raised in dysfunctional environments often suffer from a lack of self-confidence. If left unresolved (e.g., through therapy, confrontation, etc.), this lack of self-confidence can continue into adulthood. Often, these individuals unconsciously place themselves in situations in which the pattern of abuse will continue—perpetuating the belief that they are unworthy of love. In an effort to regain their senses of self-worth, some of these women shift their focus to their external selves, making their weight and appearance the center of their self-worth. Initially, as others commend these women for "taking care of themselves," they feel better about themselves.

*Make a
commitment
to work on
your inner
development.*

There are two problems with this pattern. First, the "confidence" these women have achieved isn't real; it doesn't come from within. It as an external confidence confided upon them by others, and it requires input from others to maintain. Second, the external "confidence" these women have achieved is extremely seductive, and they will go to extreme lengths to ensure others continue to recognize their efforts. It is this desire to continually solicit feedback from others that sits at the heart if an eating disorder/disordered eating. The more these women succumb to the power of this false sense of self-worth, the more desperate their efforts become to solicit positive external feedback. This, in turn, fuels the disordered eating habits and distorted thinking necessary to continue this vicious cycle.

ABUSE/DYSFUNCTION AUTOBIOGRAPHY

The *Abuse/Dysfunction Autobiography* may cause you pain and discomfort. Therefore, it is our strong recommendation that you only do this exercise if you are currently in treatment with a professional.

1. Was there any form of abuse and/or dysfunction that you experienced that was instrumental in the development of your eating disorder? If so, identify and write about these issues (be as specific as possible) that led to the development of your eating disorder. This is the beginning of your journey to healing.

_____

_____

_____

_____

_____

_____

_____

_____

_____

_____

_____

_____

_____

_____

_____

_____

_____

_____

_____

_____

_____

_____

_____

_____

_____

_____

_____

_____

We have created the following letter to nurture you in the way you were meant to be nurtured. Though you may never have the parents you always wanted you can start healing through self-parenting and self-nurturing. Allow yourself the gift of fully receiving this letter.

A Letter from your Ideal Mother

Dear _____,

I love you very much. I know you are hurting right now and I am sorry. You did not deserve the pain that was inflicted upon you. I wish I could have been the one to stop it. Hopefully it is not too late to make amends to you. I want the very best for you. You deserve it. Please give yourself the gift of healing and self-nurturing. Allow others to be there for you.

I cherish you and want the very best for you always. I want to see you happy and fulfilled. I support your healing endeavors.

Love,
Mother

Chapter Three

❧

Will I Ever be Good Enough?

The answer to the question, "Will I ever be good enough?" is a resounding YES! The unfortunate thing for many of you, however, is that throughout your lives you have either been given verbal messages or been treated by others in a way that made you feel you weren't good enough. This, in turn, led you to feel you were less than or inferior to others.

A perfect example of the feeling of never being "good enough" is seen in the modeling industry. We know our society is in trouble when even models don't measure up to the pictures of themselves. The airbrushing, touch-ups, taping, and lighting the photographers use are designed to make their pictures look better than the models look in real life. We know that models are beautiful, yet no one, not even the models themselves, can measure up to the images that bombard us daily about the perfect body. It's all just smoke and mirrors.

The concept that a very slender body is "ideal" is not new, and it is worth repeating Smolak's study from 1996 that indicated most fashion models are thinner than 98 percent of American women. This creates unrealistic expectations. It is no wonder that 80 percent of American women are dissatisfied with their appearance (Smolak, 1996). They are attempting to achieve a body type that can only be achieved through digital enhancement—not real life.

THE PERFECTIONISM TRAP

Perfectionism is a trap to which many people fall victim, and people with poor body images are particularly susceptible to the perfectionism trap. An internal striving for perfection and/or the expectations of another for us to be perfect sets the stage for feeling less-than or "not good enough." This is especially tragic when you consider the fact that there is no such thing as perfection. And because of this, if perfection is our goal, we are striving to achieve something that isn't real.

The perfectionism trap manifests itself in many different ways for different people, and it begins from two different starting points: either internal (self-inflicted) or external (expectations of others). Often the perfectionism trap begins externally and is then internalized; that is, the beliefs and expectations of others become our own.

CASE STUDY (SARA)

The external cues of perfectionism often come from family members and may begin very early in life. Take Sara, for example. The only time she received praise from her parents was when she did something fantastic. For instance, she was praised if she got "As" on her report card, but not if she got "Bs". She was praised if she got on the honor roll, but not if she was on the principal's list. Her parents often told her she was chubby, and they would give her tremendous encouragement and praise if she lost weight. These statements and behaviors left Sara feeling that if she was not perfect (i.e., thin, getting straight "As," and getting on the honor roll), her parents would not love her, nor would anybody else.

This taught Sara that her parent's love was conditional; it depended on her fulfilling their expectations. Sara's exposure to these beliefs and expectations for so many years led her to adopt them as her own. By the time Sara reached adolescence, she was diagnosed with anorexia nervosa.

EXPECTATIONS: MINE, YOURS, AND OURS

The following exercise is designed to help you identify the difference between the expectations you have set for yourself and those that have been set by other people. It is the first step in setting goals for your success as you strive to conquer your disordered eating/eating disorder.

1. What expectations do you have for yourself in all areas of your life? (school, family, career) Be specific.

School Expectations:

_____
_____
_____
_____
_____
_____
_____
_____
_____

_____
_____

Family Expectations:

_____
_____
_____
_____
_____
_____
_____
_____
_____

Career Expectations:

_____
_____
_____
_____
_____
_____
_____
_____
_____

2. Take a good look at the expectations you have listed. Are they realistic? Which ones aren't realistic?

_____
_____
_____
_____
_____
_____
_____
_____

3. If any of your expectations are unrealistic, change them into something that is possible to achieve. Use the following as an example:

Unrealistic Expectation: "I must get an 'A' in every class."

Realistic Expectation: "I will give my best effort in school and some days may be better than others, and that is OK."

Unrealistic Expectation #1:

_____

_____

Realistic Expectation #1:

_____

_____

Unrealistic Expectation #2:

_____

_____

Realistic Expectation #2:

_____

_____

Unrealistic Expectation #3:

_____

_____

Realistic Expectation #3:

_____

_____

Perfectionism is a big smokescreen. It keeps us focused on our outside selves, avoiding our real problems and insecurities. As long as people continue to strive for perfection, staying focused on the outside and avoiding dealing with the real problems, they will remain unfulfilled and unhappy. Perfectionism is truly one of the most powerful forms of self-sabotage because it is unobtainable. Do not fool yourselves into thinking, "But I am different; I can achieve perfection,"—you can't. And that is absolutely OK. The secret is learning to love the person you are—not the person you want to be.

The key to abandoning perfection as our primary objective lies in allowing ourselves to make mistakes. Everybody makes mistakes. The difference between the perfectionist and the rest of the world is: The rest of the world learns from their mistakes and moves on; the perfectionist wallows in the mistake. Instead of taking an objective look at her failure and trying to figure out why it happened and how to avoid it the next time the situation presents itself, the perfectionist chooses to avoid the situation all together. For example, an anorexic (a textbook perfectionist because of her focus on attaining the "ideal" weight) who attends a birthday party and allows herself to eat a piece of birthday cake sees enjoying the cake as a failure. Rather than allowing herself to enjoy the cake, the anorexic thinks, "Cake will make me fat. I shouldn't have had that piece of cake. If I didn't come to this party, I wouldn't have eaten the cake. I won't go to anymore parties."

We can create a positive outcome by seeking out the important information we can learn from the mistake instead of criticizing ourselves for making the mistake. We must avoid negative self-talk. We need to learn to laugh at ourselves. Humor has a way of dissipating our embarrassment when we make a mistake. In the above example, the reasonable person would have concluded, "One piece of cake isn't going to kill me," and enjoyed herself.

MY PERCEPTION OF MYSELF VS. OTHERS' PERCEPTION OF ME

As stated earlier, the perfectionism trap basically grows out of an internal (self-perception) and/or out of external (another's perception) of the type of person we should be. This difference in perception is important to explore because the reality is we cannot change the way others perceive us, but we can change the way we perceive ourselves.

We often see ourselves in a very different way than others see us, partly because we are often much more critical of ourselves than others are. Sometimes, the perceptions we have of ourselves are distorted, creating in us additional confusion about ourselves.

Below is an interesting activity that demonstrates the difference between how we perceive ourselves and how others perceive us. After completing this exercise you will have a better understanding of how you and others see you.

Animal/Color Exercise

1. Think of your favorite type of animal and write it in the space provided. Then write down three words (adjectives) that describe that animal.

Animal: _____

Descriptors: _____,_____,_____

2. Choose your favorite color; the first color that pops into your head. Jot it down in the space provided, along with three words (adjectives) that describe the color.

Color:_____

Descriptors: _____, _____, _____

The words you chose to describe the animal symbolize the way you view yourself. The descriptors you chose to describe the color symbolize how others perceive you.

The two perceptions may coincide or oppose one another. It may be interesting to take a few moments to elaborate on the differences and/or similarities you discovered through the animal/color personality profile activity. Is there a gap between the way you perceive yourself and the way others perceive you? If so, try to narrow the gap. Spend the next week making a conscious effort to demonstrate to yourself and others the newfound, positive characteristics you possess.

3. Are the perceptions you have of yourself and those possessed by others similar or opposite of one another?

_____

_____

4. What can you do to make the perceptions mirror one another more closely and create positive change?

_____

_____

_____

_____

_____

_____

_____

_____

We use the animal/color exercise as an icebreaker activity in our _Love Your Body_ Workshops. We believe it may be helpful and interesting to you if we share an example of one woman's response to this activity. (This woman gave us permission to include this case example in our book; however, we will not use her real name to ensure confidentiality.)

CASE STUDY (SUSAN)

Susan is in her early thirties and is a recovering anorexic, struggling with a negative body image. When she was asked to identify her favorite animal she chose a dog. The descriptors she used for the dog were "_large, lazy, and gentle._" Her favorite color was red. The words Susan chose to describe red were "_lively, bright, and energized._"

What does all of this mean? Susan's perception of herself is that she is a "dog" and is large, lazy, and gentle. One positive attribute found its way into the descriptors. That's a place to start. Remember the color symbolized how others perceive Susan. To Susan, others perceive her as being lively, bright, and energetic. As you can see, there is a pretty big discrepancy in the way Susan views herself and how she feels others view her.

The challenge for Susan was then to find a way to narrow the gap between these two opposing perceptions. When asked if she could understand how others may perceive her as lively, bright, and energetic, she responded with, "sometimes." She was then asked to think about what others are seeing that she doesn't allow herself to see and why she does not acknowledge these positive characteristics. She thought about it for a while, but with some journaling and processing in the group, she became aware that she negates or discounts her positive characteristics

Treat yourself with the love and kindness you give to others, and respond with a "Thank you" anytime someone compliments you.

and remains focused on what she calls her flaws. As Susan became aware of this behavior, she was able to slowly begin making changes by focusing more on her positive qualities and accepting compliments made by others.

THE DREADED MIRROR: BE MY FRIEND, NOT MY ENEMY

As you practice accepting compliments from others, practice complimenting yourself. A useful tool to use in complimenting yourself is the mirror. The mirror can be an evil enemy to somebody with a negative body image. We've heard many women say it is as though the mirror spews out negative, critical remarks to them about their bodies. However, what these women fail to recognize is that it isn't the mirror telling them these awful things about their bodies; it's them.

Negative thinking lies at the heart of our distorted body images and destructive behavior. The secret is learning how to confront these negative thoughts and seeing just how untrue they really are. To create healing and enhancement of one's body image, it is imperative to first stop talking to yourself in a negative manner, and second, replace these negative, distorted thoughts with positive, loving statements about you and your body.

MIRROR WORK WITH MY BODY

Mirror Work with My Body is a two-fold exercise. First, it allows you to address the negative thoughts you have about your body. And second, it allows you to address the negative things you tell yourself in general. The first part of this exercise will focus just on the body, whereas the second part will be overall affirmation work.

Take 10-15 minutes to stand in front of a full-length mirror. Beginning at your feet, and while looking at each body part, say a positive statement about each body part—and why you like it. The "why" part of the affirmation is important. It makes the affirmation more real and the exercise as a whole less robotic. If you prefer, it may be helpful to first write a positive statement for each body part in the space provided below. After you have written a positive statement about each body part (and don't forget the why), go to the mirror to affirm your body.

*Part I:
Affirming
My Body*

1. Feet:_____
_____

2. Calves:_____
_____

3. Thighs:_____
_____

4. Hips:_____
_____

5. Genitals:_____
_____

6. Buttocks:_____
_____

7. Abdomen:_____
_____

8. Breasts:_____
_____

9. Hands:_____
_____

10. Arms:_____
_____

11. Shoulders:_____
_____

12. Back:_____
_____

13. Neck:_____
_____

14. Face:_____
_____

15. Hair:_____
_____

The second part of the mirror work exercise is to positively affirm your *self* by using "I" statements. Make these statements aloud while standing in front of the mirror and making eye contact with yourself. You may be asking, "What is a positive affirmation?" Basically, a positive affirmation is a statement about yourself that is said in a positive manner and begins with the word, "I." For example, "I am attractive." "I am intelligent."

Now, it is your turn. List 10 positive affirmations about your *self* in the spaces provided below, then say them to yourself in the mirror. If you have difficulty thinking of 10 affirmations, think of positive things a good friend would say about you if they were asked to describe you. If you can think of more than 10, write them down. The more the merrier.

1. I _____
_____

2. I _____
_____

3. I _____
_____

4. I _____
_____

5. I _____
_____

Part II:
Affirming
My Whole Self
In the Mirror

6. I I _____
_____

7. I I _____
_____

8. I I _____
_____

9. I I _____
_____

10. I I _____
_____

This exercise is often difficult at first; however, if you keep at it, it will get easier. Consistency is important. If you keep at it, you will most likely notice a difference in how you feel about your body

Add one new affirmation to your list each week. Make a commitment to yourself to do Parts 1 and 2 of this exercise every day for 30 days. Remember, consistency is the key. Take some time to document or make a mental note to yourself as to whether you feel any different about your body and yourself as a whole at the end of the 30 days.

Affirmation work is designed to increase self-acceptance. It is our hope that as you completed the above exercise you were able to see the difference between fantasy thinking and setting realistic expectations about your body. Unrealistic expectations can result in self-sabotage. Another way to sabotage recovery is through incongruent action. When your values are not in alignment with your behaviors, sabotage occurs. This results in a failure to achieve the goal/task you set out to accomplish. The next section further explores the correlation between your values and your behaviors.

*Look in the
mirror and
say, "I am
beautiful!"*

THE VALUES/BEHAVIOR CORRELATION

We all have a core set of values. These are our inner beliefs that we see as extremely important. Some people rate honesty in their top five values. They would rather know the truth than a fabricated story, even if that meant their feelings could get hurt. Some people value reliability. They are attracted to others who are reliable. It is these core values that drive us; they make us do the things we do. However, whenever one of our core values is out of line with our actions, it causes us discomfort.

Take, for example, the emphasis many of us place on health and fitness. It is safe to say that the majority of people recognize the importance of maintaining a healthy lifestyle. And while we live in a society that is certainly conscious of the importance of exercise and cooking meals, we leave very little time for these activities. Most of us are too busy putting in 60-hour workweeks, taking our kids to and from their seemingly endless extracurricular activities, or driving to our next big social event. This places many of us, particularly those who strive for perfection, in a quandary.

There is a price to pay when we value something but do not act accordingly. When we do not follow through on living in accordance with our values, we sabotage ourselves. For example, if we value honesty but engage in dishonest behaviors, we pay the price of guilt. If we value fairness, yet cheat, we are angry at, and disappointed in, ourselves. The same holds true for health and fitness. If we value being healthy but don't exercise and don't eat right, we pay the price with poor health.

Most of us do not feel very good about ourselves when we betray our core values, and it creates a negative feedback loop. Guilt, anger, depression, and frustration are not motivators. Destructive emotions tend to take away our motivation. Why? Because when we feel bad about ourselves, we tend to engage in negative, punishing behaviors, such as overeating, purging, negative self-talk, restriction of food, and so forth. These negative feelings lead us right back into the negative behaviors, creating a negative feedback loop that altogether bypasses our values. On the other hand, when we take proper action to promote our values it raises self-esteem, builds character, and enhances recovery.

Let's take a look at the following diagrams that illustrate both the positive and the negative outcomes of the *Values/Behavior Correlation*.

Figure 3.1: Values/Behavior Correlation (Positive Outcome)

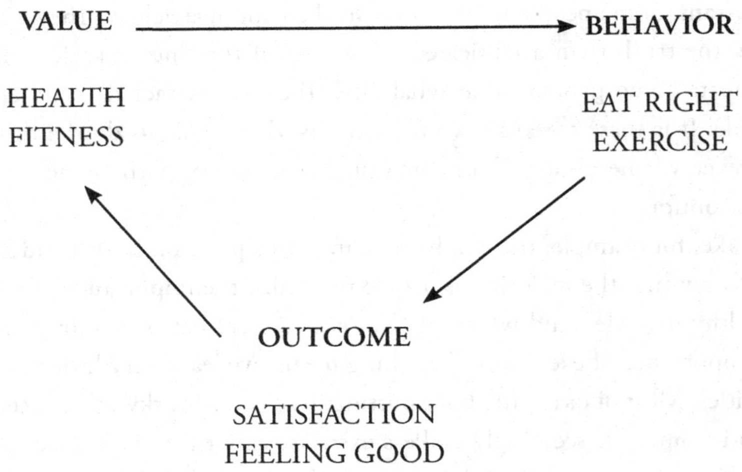

VALUE ————————————▶ BEHAVIOR

HEALTH   EAT RIGHT
FITNESS   EXERCISE

OUTCOME

SATISFACTION
FEELING GOOD

Figure 3.2: Values/Behavior Correlation (Negative Outcome)

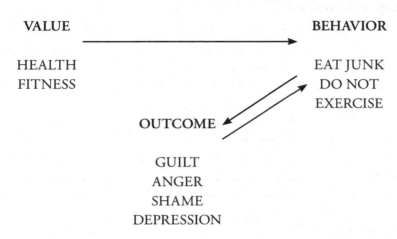

When we value something and follow through on it we feel good, and feeling good is motivating and nurturing. Positive action and nurturing reinforce the behavior that corresponds to the value. On the other hand, when our behavior is counter to our values, the outcome is negative: We feel guilty, angry, depressed, and/or disappointed in ourselves.

SHINING THE LIGHT ON SABOTAGE

The following exercise is designed to align your values and behaviors to create a successful recovery.

1. How do you sabotage yourself? List the value you desire and what you do to sabotage accomplishing that value. Remember to be as specific as possible. Use the following as an example.

Value: Fit Body
Sabotaging Behavior: Don't make time for exercise. Make poor food choices.

Value #1:_____

_____

Sabotaging Behavior #1:_____
_____

Value #2:_____
_____

Sabotaging Behavior #2:_____
_____

Value #3:_____
_____

Sabotaging Behavior #3:_____
_____

Value #4:_____
_____

Sabotaging Behavior #4:_____
_____

Value #5:_____
_____

Sabotaging Behavior #5:_____
_____

2. List these values again and now list healthy behaviors you are willing to engage in to achieve each value. Use the following as an example.

Value: Fit Body
Healthy Behavior: I will do 20 minutes of exercise four times per week. I will eat more balanced throughout the day, making an effort to eat more fruits and vegetables. I am committed to making healthier food choices without going overboard.

Be true to yourself by backing up your values with the appropriate behaviors.

Value #1:_____

_____

Healthy Behavior #1:_____

_____

Value #2:_____

_____

Healthy Behavior #2:_____

_____

Value #3:_____

_____

Healthy Behavior #3:_____

_____

Value #4:_____

_____

Healthy Behavior #4:_____

_____

Value #5:_____

_____

Healthy Behavior #5:_____

_____

Chapter Four

❧

Obstacles to Change

Change is a choice. Most of us are creatures of habit and like being so. For many people the concept, or even the idea, of change is scary. It can bring about feelings of fear and anxiety, even when the change is positive.

Change brings a foreign element – something different – into our lives. It does not matter what that foreign element is, such as a new job, a baby, or the break-up of a relationship. All we know is that something is different, and therefore out of the norm, which can be uncomfortable. Often, to escape feeling uncomfortable, we avoid addressing the foreign element in order to evade the feelings associated with it. The bottom line is this, in the beginning, doing something different can be awkward and anxiety producing. However, we must allow ourselves to feel and experience the anxiety in order to move forward. Let's look at a case example.

Case Study (Lori)

There was a woman whom we shall call Lori. Lori had experienced a great deal of change in her life over a six-month period. Upon entering therapy she stated she was feeling lost, confused, extremely overwhelmed, and simply out of control of her life. She had graduated from a four-year university in June, was married in August, moved into a new home in September, and was having difficulty finding a permanent position in a teaching career, which she had gone to school for. This background on Lori helps us to understand where her feelings of being overwhelmed and out of control were coming from. The changes in her life were tremendous and all of them happened in a short period of time. The more out of control Lori felt, the more rigid she became with her food. She felt she had little or no control over the many events taking place in her life; however, the one aspect she did have control over was her food and eating behavior.

Lori's Rigid Food Plan

Lori had been keeping herself on a very rigid food plan for several years. Here is an example of a typical day of nutrition for Lori:

Breakfast: Piece of fruit, usually banana or apple - small in size. (This meal was often skipped altogether.)

Lunch: Small green leafy salad (no dressing) with three saltine crackers.

Dinner: Small amount of brown rice, lots of vegetables (spinach, green beans, broccoli, cauliflower).

Snack: Yogurt (light).

For Lori to make changes in her "food plan," she had to allow herself to experience the feelings that come along with change; yet, instead of this she was running from them to feel more "comfortable." This kept her stuck, doing the same old thing. The control she thought she had over her food was only pseudo-control. Instead, it was the food and behaviors related to eating that had control over Lori; she did not have control over them. In order for Lori to take control she needs to practice her new healthy behaviors until she becomes comfortable with them and they become part of her status quo.

Case Study (Kathy)

Kathy is a fifty-three year old married woman with three grown children. She has successfully lost weight several times, only to regain it back. She knows she has to change her life, but feels overwhelmed to do so. Kathy turns to food to numb her feelings. She is bored, stuck, and depressed. Kathy's physician has told her she needs to lose twenty-five pounds for health reasons. This seems impossible, because of her numerous failed diet attempts. Kathy expresses feeling more depressed about this and her over-eating has escalated.

Kathy's Food Plan

Kathy, being a chronic dieter, either restricts or over-indulges. Currently, she is in a binge-cycle. The following is an example of a typical day of eating for Kathy:

Breakfast: 1 bowl of bran cereal with nonfat milk, a small apple, and 1 cup of coffee.

Snack: 2 cinnamon rice cakes.

Lunch: Chinese chicken salad with dressing on the side and ice tea.

Snack: 2 large chocolate chip cookies (while shopping at the mall).

Snack: Grab bag size of potato chips (while waiting for husband to come home and go out for dinner).

Dinner: 2 baskets of chips and salsa, chicken tostada, and a margarita (restaurant).

Snack: Chocolate cake and vanilla ice cream (leftover birthday cake and ice cream).

At first glance Kathy's food plan looks good. She starts the morning off with a small healthy breakfast, followed by a midmorning snack and a healthy lunch. On the outside her choices look healthy. On the inside however, there is a growing sense of deprivation. This interferes with her ability to sustain healthy eating habits. This inner struggle opens the door to bingeing. The bingeing behavior is enticing for two reasons. First, Kathy is able to escape the feelings of deprivation, and second it is providing an unhealthy way to self-nurture. In order for Kathy to change this destructive cycle, she must work through the negative feelings and nurture herself in a healthy way not related to food (See Chapter 7 section on, *Nurturing Activities*).

The following exercise, *The Role of Food in Your Life*, is to gain awareness of how you use food for reasons other than satisfying physical hunger.

The Role of Food in Your Life

1. Have you ever used food in order to feel like you have some sense of control of your life?

2. If so, how did the pattern begin, and what did it progress to?

_____

_____

_____

_____

_____

_____

_____

_____

_____

_____

_____

Did you find that the role of food in your life has progressed in a negative way? Is food covering up feelings of sadness, anger, hurt, etc.? When you control your food, does it make you feel better temporarily? Has controlling your food become a trap because your feelings are still unresolved? Most likely the answers to these questions are "yes". For this reason, the _Food Log_ will address your eating behavior in relation to your thoughts and feelings.

FOOD LOG

Log your food for one week in order to get a clearer picture about your struggle with unbalanced eating. It may be either is rigid or over-indulgent. It is helpful to become aware of any eating behavior linked to an emotional reaction. Emotions stem from thoughts, therefore if you can change the way you think, you can change the way you feel. For this reason, document both your feelings and your thoughts right before and during meals.

Day 1

Time	What you ate?	How much? (approx.)	Feelings	Thoughts

Day 2

Time	What you ate?	How much? (approx.)	Feelings	Thoughts

Day 3

Time	What you ate?	How much? (approx.)	Feelings	Thoughts

Day 4

Time	What you ate?	How much? (approx.)	Feelings	Thoughts

Day 5

Time	What you ate?	How much? (approx.)	Feelings	Thoughts

Day 6

Time	What you ate?	How much? (approx.)	Feelings	Thoughts

Day 7

Time	What you ate?	How much? (approx.)	Feelings	Thoughts

1. Did you see a pattern in your eating in regard to feelings, instead of physical hunger?

_____

_____

2. If so, identify the feelings that tend to trigger emotional eating. For example, many people eat out of boredom.

_____

_____

_____

_____

3. Make a list of activities you can do, instead of turning to food, to nurture yourself when your emotions take over. If you need help, look at the list of _Nurturing Activities_ in Chapter 7.

_____

_____

_____

_____

_____

_____

_____

_____

ॐ

Remain an active participant in your recovery at all times.

TAKE AN ACTIVE ROLE IN CREATING CHANGE

Creating change in our lives requires that we play an active role. We make a commitment to ourselves to keep working hard at making our body image more positive, even if we feel uncomfortable at times, or even if the activities in the book stir up feelings we have been trying to avoid. You are worth it! The results are phenomenal! Even doing something that seems easy, such as positive self-talk, can feel uncomfortable and that discomfort or awkwardness causes many people to stop. Don't let the negativity win; it has already taken up too much of your valuable time and energy.

A helpful technique to use when anxiety, or any other uncomfortable feeling, surfaces is to engage in slow, deep breathing to calm yourself down. When you get anxious, everything constricts, cutting off the amount of oxygen getting into your bloodstream. You can reduce your anxiety by increasing the amount of oxygen you are breathing in.

Another valuable tool is to release your thoughts and feelings by journaling. Remember, your negative feelings have much more power and intensity when you hold them inside.

Relaxation Technique

To assist you in decreasing your anxiety and to help you relax, the following is a simple relaxation exercise with guided imagery for you to learn and practice.

1. Write about a place that creates a sense of peace and serenity for you. This place can be either real or imagined. It is a place just for you, so have fun with it. Be as specific as possible. Using all your senses, write down all the details you can think of, in order to make it very real in your mind when doing the relaxation exercise.

_____

_____

_____

_____

_____

_____

_____

_____

_____

_____

Now it's time to practice the relaxation exercise.

Sit comfortably in your chair with both feet on the floor. Close your eyes and begin to take deep, slow breaths, allowing your body to relax. As you exhale, feel any tension or stress you may have in your body exit through your fingertips and toes. Continue to breathe slowly and deeply throughout the guided imagery exercise. Good. Your body is feeling more and more relaxed.

Visualize a soft pink fog entering your body with every breath (If there is another color that provides a deep sense of calm and peace use that color instead). This pink fog carries with it a sense of calm, positive, healing energy. See this comforting pink entity move through and around your head, relaxing all the muscles in your face and head... Taking away any negative or distracting thoughts in your mind... Move the pink oxygen down your neck, allowing time for the oxygen to penetrate any stress you hold in your neck and shoulders – releasing all the tension as your muscles become completely relaxed... Continue to move the pink fog down to your chest... your upper back... your lower back releasing all the muscle tension... See the pink healing force of the oxygen in your internal organs, your heart... your lungs... your kidneys... and your stomach... bringing healing and peace to these areas... Stay here awhile to allow the healing energy to work through all your internal organs... Now, move to your pelvic region... your thighs... your calves... your ankles... your feet... and your toes...

Now, see your entire body filled with the pink healing oxygen... it is both throughout your body and surrounding your body like a warm cozy blanket... Allow the pink healing force to be a filter and allow only the positive in and repel all the negative... See yourself with this healing force everyday and know you can always utilize its power and positive energy whenever you feel stressed, overwhelmed, or need to reenergize... It's always there for you... simply close your eyes, take deep, slow breaths, and bring forth the image of your pink healing oxygen...

Now that your body and mind are relaxed go to your safe, peaceful place that you have created for yourself... Maybe it is the beach at sunset... the mountains... or sitting by a lake... wherever your special place is, see yourself there now... Give yourself a moment to experience the peace and serenity this place gives to you... inhale the peace and calm this place provides for you so you can take it with you... This place is always available to you, at any time... You created it... Whenever you need peace or calming, just close your eyes and put yourself in your safe, serene place... it is there just for you. Take in a few more deep breaths, inhaling this sense of calm to bring back with you, as you bring your awareness back into the room you are presently in. Count back from 5 to 1. When you are ready and feel comfortable you may open your eyes. You will feel relaxed and refreshed throughout the rest of the day... 5,4,3,2,1.

Relaxation allows you to be receptive to change.

Journaling demonstrates how you are taking an active stance in the process of your change and healing. You cannot be an innocent bystander in this process, it just doesn't work. Verbally make a contract with yourself that you will do whatever it takes to create a positive body image. As an active participant in your recovery process, journal in the space provided your experience doing the relaxation exercise above.

Use the space below to journal the thoughts and feelings you experienced during the relaxation exercise.

_____

_____

_____

_____

_____

_____

MY ROAD TO RECOVERY

Many women have been living with, and still carry around, a negative body image for many years. Negative feelings are a tremendous burden and take a significant toll on you physically, mentally, emotionally and spiritually. Negativity about anything takes the focus off the positive, draining one's energy. In designing your own road to recovery, you must first figure out your "road blocks." Everybody's road to recovery is different. This next exercise may be quite a challenge for some of you, but stick with it. There is no right or wrong way to do the following exercise, so have fun and be creative. You may come to some fascinating realizations you were unaware of previously.

First, take a few minutes to clear your mind of any "brain traffic." Simply close your eyes and begin to breathe slowly and deeply, allowing your mind and body to relax. Focus on your breathing, notice how deep and slow your breathing is and the soothing effect that deep and slow breathing is having on your body. Fully clear out any thoughts in your mind (e.g., grocery list, errands to run, etc.) Continue to focus on your breathing, allowing yourself to feel more and more relaxed...

Now, see yourself walking down a road or path... Pay close attention to the

PART I:
_Uncovering the
Obstacles_

details around you... Are there any noticeable landmarks you are passing? Is anybody else on this road? Is this road well traveled? Is it one lane, many lanes, or isolated in the country? Are there any houses, buildings, trees, bushes, or fences that line this road? What is the texture of the road? Is the road smooth or bumpy, with lots of potholes and oil slicks? Again, just take a few minutes to fully notice the environment around you... This road is the path to recovery from your negative body image; therefore, is has a great deal of valuable information to share with you. The details are important!

At this time, focus on any object that presents itself as an obstacle... This may be a road block... a dead-end street... potholes... oil slicks... a road under construction... Whatever the obstacle is, focus on it... Ask this obstacle what important information it has to share with you on the road to healing your body image issues... There may be more than one obstacle... The obstacle(s) are often items that you must address or process in order to create a more positive body image for yourself... If you come across more than one "road block," approach it as you did the first obstacle and ask it to tell you what it represents and how you can resolve that issue... Repeat this step until all obstacles have been confronted... As you confront each obstacle, make a mental note of the important information it has for you...

When you have confronted and communicated with each obstacle, redirect your focus back to your breathing and allow your mind and body to feel relaxed. Take as much time as you need to re-center yourself to your surroundings (e.g., "I'm in my room sitting on my bed," "I'm in the living room sitting on the couch," etc). When you have opened your eyes, draw the road you visualized and any obstacles you encountered. Make sure you label all the obstacles and write down the messages they had for you in regards to healing your body image. Complete this in the space provided.

Draw a picture of your road with the obstacles.

Great, you've finished part one of this exercise! Now, it's time to *recreate* your road to recovery. This part is really exciting in that you have the power to create your own safety zones, remove or change the obstacles, and create healing in your life. Make sure you complete part two of the *Road to Recovery* exercise. If you uncover the obstacles to your success without recreating your road, your life will not change.

Once again, close your eyes and take in slow, deep breaths, allowing your mind and body to fully relax. Clear your mind of any "brain traffic" so you may focus just on this exercise. Now, place yourself back on your path or road, remembering all of its details… Continue walking until you reach the first obstacle… Now create a way to get around, through, or over the obstacle… For example, if the obstacle is an oil slick, see yourself pour sand over it to make it possible for you to walk over it… If you see a total break in the road filled with water, making it impossible for you to continue, place a small bridge over the water, connecting the two parts of the road so you can continue… No obstacle has the power to immobilize you… Continue to defeat each obstacle until you have conquered them all…

Now, see yourself at a positive, nurturing place on this road… Create a scene that is pleasurable, joyful, loving, and nurturing… Maybe you see lots of colorful flowers lining a smoothly paved road… If the sun is shining, feel the warmth of the sun on your BEAUTIFUL body… Allow yourself to feel the joy, love, and encouragement surrounding you… Visualize embracing yourself and giving yourself a heartfelt hug… Sit with this image for a few moments… Tell yourself you are beautiful and unique… Continue to experience the positive overflow of acceptance and newfound love for your body… As you allow yourself to remain in this positive space, become reconnected to your surrounding environment, becoming fully aware of where you are (e.g., bedroom, living room, etc.). Now, it's time to draw your new road to recovery, with conquered obstacles and all. To capture your mental image, be sure to include as many details as you can.

PART II: My Healing Road to Recovery

Draw your new road to recovery.

The purpose of the previous exercise was to design your road to recovery. Now that your map is complete, it is your task to follow it.

Chapter Five

&

Choosing a Healthy
Body Image

Now that you have identified the obstacles that have prevented you from accepting your body, it is time to create a healthy body image. By choosing a healthy body image, you increase your self-esteem. We have developed *Eleven Ways to Learn to Love Your Body* as concrete steps to begin creating your healthy body image.

ELEVEN WAYS TO LEARN TO LOVE YOUR BODY

ONE: DON'T COMPARE

When we compare ourselves to others we always lose. The realities of our own looks, as well as everyone else's, don't even matter. When we look at others, we seem to see how perfect they are. When we look at ourselves, we only see our own imperfections. We feel we can never measure up, no matter what. Society and popular culture only make matters worse by worshipping an elusive fantasy body that only a few women on earth could ever naturally attain. By avoiding comparisons to others, we save ourselves lots of grief and can work towards making the body God gave us the best it can be.

Let go of the internal critic. Document how many times you compare yourself to others this week. First write down the critical thoughts, either about yourself or someone else, and then rewrite them into more positive statements.

Day 1

Number of critical thoughts when comparing myself to others:

_____

_____

My critical thoughts:

_____

_____

_____

_____

_____

Rewrite the critical thoughts into more positive statements:

_____

Day 2

Number of critical thoughts when comparing myself to others:

_____

My critical thoughts:

_____

Rewrite the critical thoughts into more positive statements:

_____

_____
_____
_____
_____
_____
_____
_____
_____
_____

Day 3

Number of critical thoughts when comparing myself to others:
_____
_____

My critical thoughts:
_____
_____
_____
_____
_____
_____
_____
_____
_____

Rewrite the critical thoughts into more positive statements:
_____
_____
_____
_____
_____
_____
_____
_____
_____

Day 4

Number of critical thoughts when comparing myself to others:

_____

_____

My critical thoughts:

_____

_____

_____

_____

_____

_____

_____

_____

Rewrite the critical thoughts into more positive statements.

_____

_____

_____

_____

_____

_____

_____

_____

_____

Day 5

Number of critical thoughts when comparing myself to others:

_____

_____

My critical thoughts:

_____

_____

_____
_____
_____
_____
_____
_____
_____
_____

Rewrite the critical thoughts into more positive statements.

_____
_____
_____
_____
_____
_____
_____
_____
_____

Day 6

Number of critical thoughts when comparing myself to others:

_____
_____

My critical thoughts:

_____
_____
_____
_____
_____
_____
_____
_____

Rewrite the critical thoughts into more positive statements.

_____

_____

_____

_____

_____

_____

_____

_____

_____

_____

Day 7

Number of critical thoughts when comparing myself to others:

_____

_____

My critical thoughts:

_____

_____

_____

_____

_____

_____

_____

_____

_____

Rewrite the critical thoughts into more positive statements.

_____

_____

_____

_____

_____

_____

_____

_____

Congratulations! By changing your critical thoughts into positive statements, you have begun to learn to accept yourself and not compare yourself to others.

Two: Focus on Your Accomplishments

Instead of nit-picking your body, try to focus on your positive traits. Are you loving, kind, and considerate? Do you visit your grandmother regularly? Do you get good grades? Are you a wonderful mother? Spouse? Are you known for the fun parities you throw? Can you draw? We all have talents and attributes that make us wonderful human beings. So what if your thighs are not pencil thin? You make a difference in the world, and that is what really matters!

Victory Journal

In order to focus on your accomplishments, let's begin a *Victory Journal*. Either decorate a journal to reflect your unique personality or go out and purchase a new one. This journal will only be used for your victories. At the end of each day, make a list of everything you have accomplished. Victories come in all shapes and sizes. Some are big, such as confronting a person who has done something upsetting to you; and others, like adding 5 minutes more to your exercise routine, are small. Too often we focus on what we are doing wrong, instead of what we are doing right. The important thing to remember is to give yourself credit for the positive strides you take every single day. In the space below, list your accomplishments from over the past week. Then, go out and create your *Victory Journal!*

My Accomplishments:

_____

_____

_____

_____

_____

_____

Three: Learn to Take a Compliment

Many of us dream of looking perfect. We want to be beautiful and have others stop and notice us. Yet, when someone gives us a compliment such as, "You look great in that dress," we react by saying something like, "This old thing!" The very thing we wish for – recognition – we brush off. Practice saying "thank you" with confidence when someone gives you compliment. Don't over analyze or judge the giver; instead, let the compliment soak in and allow yourself to feel really good. A compliment is a verbal gift someone is giving to you. Be a gracious recipient, instead of giving the gift back by discounting it.

Make an effort to notice the positive statements people say to you. Write them down and then same them aloud in the mirror.

Four: Self-Talk

Pay attention to the chatter that goes on in your head. Are you saying nice thing to yourself? Are you being complimentary of your body? Are you using words of encouragement? Chances are you answered "no" to these questions. Many of us go around with a negative tape recorder playing in our head all day long.

When we stop and listen, we hear thoughts like, "Why did you do that? You are so stupid!" or "I can't believe you actually said that, it sounded so dumb!" Replace these negative thoughts with praise, such as, "What a good idea. That was a good way of handling the situation," or "That was a real accomplishment, I'm so proud!" By shifting from words of criticism to words of praise, you begin to change your life.

After you have monitored and documented the critical thoughts about yourself when you compare yourself to others, it is now time to take this one step further. Monitor the overall negative self-talk that you engage in on a daily basis. For one week, monitor and record any general negative thoughts you might have about yourself. Once you are fully aware of these thoughts, you gain the power to transform them into positive thoughts.

Day 1

My negative thoughts:

_____

_____

_____

_____

_____

_____

_____

_____

_____

Rewrite the negative thoughts into more positive statements.

_____

_____

_____

_____

_____

_____

_____

_____

Day 2

My negative thoughts:

_____
_____
_____
_____
_____
_____
_____
_____
_____
_____
_____

Rewrite the negative thoughts into more positive statements.

_____
_____
_____
_____
_____
_____
_____
_____
_____

Day 3

My negative thoughts:

_____
_____
_____
_____
_____
_____
_____
_____

Rewrite the negative thoughts into more positive statements.

_____

_____

_____

_____

_____

_____

_____

_____

Day 4

My negative thoughts:

_____

_____

_____

_____

_____

_____

_____

_____

_____

_____

Rewrite the negative thoughts into more positive statements.

_____

_____

_____

_____

_____

_____

_____

_____

Day 5

My negative thoughts:

_____
_____
_____
_____
_____
_____
_____
_____
_____
_____
_____
_____

Rewrite the negative thoughts into more positive statements.

_____
_____
_____
_____
_____
_____
_____
_____
_____
_____

Day 6

My negative thoughts:

_____
_____
_____
_____
_____
_____
_____
_____
_____
_____

Rewrite the negative thoughts into more positive statements.

_____
_____
_____
_____
_____
_____
_____
_____

Day 7

My negative thoughts:

_____
_____
_____
_____
_____
_____
_____
_____
_____
_____

Rewrite the negative thoughts into more positive statements.

_____
_____
_____
_____
_____
_____
_____

FIVE: AFFIRMATIONS

Combined with self-talk, giving yourself positive affirmations is a powerful tool to change the way you feel about your body. Find a part of your body that you like and accept as it is, such as your eyes, hair, and smile. Write an affirmation about it. For instance, "I love the way my hair shines," or "I love the way my eyes sparkle." Look at yourself in the mirror every morning and repeat your affirmations. Say them with enthusiasm! Believe them! Even if you have to "fake it till you make it." In time, you will come to believe and realize that what you are saying is true. Then move onto another body part. As you progress, you may find you have a hard time giving compliments to certain parts of your body, but continue through until you LOVE YOUR BODY! Make sure you are spending time in the mirror daily with both your body affirmations, as well as the general affirmations you wrote down in Chapter 3, *Will I Ever Be Good Enough?*

SIX: LEARN TO COMPLIMENT OTHERS

In learning to compliment others, you learn the law of reciprocity. As you give, you receive. By learning to acknowledge the good in others, you can learn to notice the good in yourself. Remember: to be loved, you must give love. To be accepting of your body, be accepting of other's bodies. Make a conscious effort to compliment somebody else at least once each day. Document the compliments you make to others for one week. This will help you focus on the positive.

COMPLEMENTS TO OTHERS

Day 1

_____

_____

Day 2

_____

_____

Day 3

_____

_____

Day 4

_____

_____

Day 5

_____

_____

Day 6

_____

_____

Day 7

_____

_____

❧

When you quiet your inner-critic and focus on positive thoughts, you are well on your way to recovery

Seven: Focus on the Positives

Hating the body can become a bad habit. All our negative feelings are instantly transferred to the body. Instead of dealing with the problems that create negative feelings, we just shove these feelings deep inside and end up hating ourselves more and more. Learning to focus on the positives gives you a whole different perspective. It allows you to see the world half-full, instead of half-empty. Focus on the good in your life. Admire the beauty of a sunset, take a walk along the water's edge, or stop and smell the roses. Begin to focus and see the good in your body. It gets you where you are going. It is a faithful companion. By focusing on the positive we begin to heal our negative body image. Refer back to your affirmations in Chapter 3 *Will I Ever be Good Enough?* Do you see a trend here?

EIGHT: STOP FANTASY THINKING

Do you ever hear yourself saying, "If I'd just lose 10 pounds I'd be happy," or "If I had thinner thighs I'd be asked out more." Stop these thoughts now! That is fantasy thinking. The truth is that there is room for all shapes and sizes in this world. People are attracted to others for a variety of reasons. Yes, sometimes attraction has to do with body, but that might be a smile or overall appearance. Others are attracted to others based on the energy they give off, or their laugh, or because they are funny. Your body is not the reason you are miserable. You were miserable first and then took it out on your body. Now get on with your life. Be loving and you will attract loving people. While doing your affirmation work this week, try rubbing your favorite scented lotion on your body at the same time you are affirming your body. This is a kind and nurturing act, demonstrating love and respect for your body.

NINE: HEAL YOUR RELATIONSHIP WITH FOOD

If you are always afraid of what food will do to your body, you are afraid of food. Will you become huge? Will you start eating and never stop? Will you go hungry? Will you be stuffed? Will you explode? To heal your relationship with food, start by selecting a food which is slightly out of your safe zone and is only a little bit challenging. Over the next week, try to challenge yourself on three different occasions with slightly challenging foods. After each new food adventure, journal your thoughts and feelings about the experience and remember: it is only food. Sit in a quiet room and take a few deep breaths. Now eat that food. Stop any negative thoughts that enter your mind. Replace those thoughts with positive ones and say affirmations. Learn to enjoy the taste of food.

Food #1:

_____

_____

My experience:

_____

_____

_____
_____
_____
_____

Food #2:
_____
_____

My experience:
_____
_____
_____
_____
_____

Food #3:
_____
_____

My experience:

On your healing journey, make an effort to continue to challenge yourself with food choices.

_____
_____
_____
_____
_____
_____

TEN: BODY MOVEMENT

The body was designed to move. To walk, run, jump, and dance are normal activities. By reconnecting yourself to your body, you might be amazed at how incredible it really is. Yoga is a great way to reconnect with your body. It is a noncompetitive, gentle, stretching program that will relax you and make your body feel wonderful. If you do not want a structured program and hate the gym, go for a walk. A walk in nature is especially comforting and nature is non-judgmental.

Experience how your body feels on your walks. Be aware of your breathing. Do not force yourself to exercise; allow yourself the opportunity to move. Create a list of activities you will commit to trying in finding adventurous ways to get your body in motion. Remember: for many people, variety is key to maintaining fun so that your activities do not become boring. Make a commitment to try at least two of these activities over the next week.

FUN PHYSICAL ACTIVITIES

1._____

2._____

3._____

4._____

5._____

6._____

7._____

8._____

9._____

10._____

ELEVEN: SUPPORT

The struggle to heal your negative body image is an ongoing battle. It is often

When you need support, allow yourself to reach out.

wise to seek the professional help of a therapist or dietitian. There are also self-help groups available at no charge (See Appendix, *List of Eating Disorder Organizations*). Many books and articles have been written on the subjects of food and the body. Seminars are available, as well as church and temple groups. Talk to a trusted friend or relative. All of us need support. We are constantly barraged with messages about the fantasy body and are given negative messages of food and weight. It is extremely hard in our culture to have a healthy, positive body image. You need support, you deserve it!

Chapter Six

❧

The Emotional Healing Triad

The *Emotional Healing Triad* consists of three components: thinking, feeling, and nurturing behavior or activities. Our spirit lies within the very center of these components (See Figure 6.1: *The Emotional Healing Triad* diagram, below). The triad is interlinked so that when you address one component, the other two are directly affected. Since many people manage to bury their feelings so long they no longer remember what they really feel, the easiest place to start on the triad is the 'thinking' component. The way you think directly affects the way you feel and your mood, which in turn have an impact on how you act or behave.

Figure 6.1: The Emotional Healing Triad

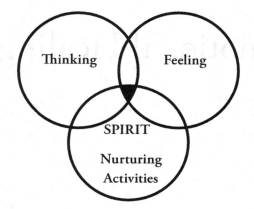

At the center where the three components intersect one another is your SPIRIT.

Because thoughts can dictate emotions, if you can change the way you think, you can change the way you feel! Therefore, the most effective way to start is by working on your way of thinking. It is often difficult for people to make the shift from negative to positive thinking and behavior, especially for people who were raised in families where there was a lot of chaos and criticism. An important factor to remember is that we are all the product of our environment and upbringing, whether we like it or not. An equally important factor to remember is that we do not have to stay grounded in negativity or continue dysfunctional behaviors, even if that is what we learned growing up. In times of crisis, we often run on autopilot, meaning we revert back to behaviors that are familiar, learned, and well practiced. Growing up, our role models were the people closest to us in our daily lives and as little children we absorbed everything around us like small sponges. The significant adults, usually our parents or caretakers, modeled for us how to argue or not, treat people with respect, and show affection, hostility, or anger to others, as well as to ourselves. Displays of verbal and nonverbal communication were, and still are, very powerful in shaping our habitual behaviors. To become aware of how we behave in various situations, as well as what we are thinking and feeling requires a conscious effort. Once we become aware of these behaviors, thoughts, and emotions, we can decide what is undesirable and nonproductive for us, and work on changing. We do not have to remain stuck in the same place, recreating the same patterns that we hated so much as children.

Our thoughts, feelings, and behaviors are all interlinked; therefore, we must look at each component in the change process. Figure 6.2: *The Inter-Linking Process of Change* illustrates this interlinking relationship.

Figure 6.2: The Inter-Linking Process of Change

Changes in
Thinking

Reinforces   *Reinforces*

Changes in   Changes in
Behavior   Feelings?

Leads to

For most of us, the easiest place to start change is in the element of thinking. Our thoughts directly affect and create the way we feel, which in turn affects our behavior. The "Thought-Stopping" technique is highly effective in stopping negative thoughts. Simply "stop" yourself and verbally say "No" or "Stop" when you catch yourself thinking negative thoughts. Sometimes it can be helpful to wear a rubber band around your wrist and GENTLY snap it when you catch yourself engaging in negative thinking as a reminder.

Once you have caught yourself in the negative thinking mode, replace the negative thought with a positive one. If you find that little negative self, sitting

Use the "Thought-Stopping" technique to stop the negative thinking.

on your shoulder, trying to whisper or scream negative thoughts into your ear, simply flick it off your shoulder. Tell it you are not going to listen to its garbage anymore! The next activity will explore the "thinking" component in detail.

The following table will demonstrate in more detail the concept of the interrelation of the three components of the *Emotional Healing Triad*. One evening Marisa, who is a recovering anorexic, was clothes shopping with her friends and having a great time. She was really enjoying their company, until one of her friends remarked, "You really look great. You look so much healthier!" This was meant as a compliment; however, Marisa interpreted the comment much differently. Remember that, up until this point, Marisa was in a good mood and having a great time. Suddenly, this one comment made a significant shift in Marisa's mood. She internalized this comment as, "She thinks I've gained weight. I must look fat. I'm such a gross pig." This negative and irrational thinking led to a shift back into the harmful feelings of being fat, unattractive, hopeless, and inferior. Due to her sensitivity about her weight, she automatically and unconsciously interpreted her friend's comments as negative. Although the healthy part of her brain knew her friend was only complimenting and encouraging her, the critical part interpreted the comment as negative. The thoughts, which generated the pessimistic feelings, resulted in destructive eating behavior. After Marisa and her friends finished their shopping, they went to dinner; however, Marisa chose not to eat. She told her friends she was not hungry, even though it was now 8:00pm and she last ate at noon. Marisa is a classic example of how our thoughts, feelings, and behaviors are interrelated and affect one another. Below is a table to help you better visualize the interrelatedness of the thoughts, feelings and behaviors.

Figure 6.3: Interrelatedness of Thoughts, Feelings and Behavior

		Anorexia	Bulimia	Compulsive Overeating
Thoughts	**Feelings**	**Behavior**	**Behavior**	**Behavior**
She thinks I've gained weight.	Unattractive	Restriction	Binge/Purge	Binge
I must look fat.	Hopeless, Unattractive, Gross	Restriction	Binge/Purge	Binge

I'm such a gross pig.	Inferior, Unlovable, Disgusting	Restriction	Binge/Purge	Binge

Reality Check! It is important to revaluate your thinking when an intense feeling surfaces, in order to make sure you are being realistic. Either revaluate your perception of what another person said for clarification, or challenge the thought if it is irrational. The next section of this chapter will address distorted and irrational thoughts in more depth.

A significant part of healing is to work on changing the way you think and acknowledge your feelings. If your thoughts are self-limiting, negative, and hopeless you won't stand a chance. However, if your thoughts are upbeat and optimistic, your feelings will be too, which will allow healing to occur. In a culture so taken by a fantasy body, it is easy to slip into critical thinking mode. If you catch yourself imagining something derogatory about your body, always counter these thoughts with a positive affirmation, such as, "I am a beautiful and unique creation of God."

"I am a beautiful and unique creation of God."

Negative Thinking

Most of us can relate to finding ourselves engaged in negative thinking every now and then. However, if you have a poor body image, you probably engage in negative thinking much more frequently than someone with a positive body image. One of the frustrating things about negative thoughts (which are often distorted) is that they are frequently automatic, with one negative thought triggering the next. Because they can become automatic, your first step is to become aware of what your negative thoughts are.

Part I: Uncover Your Negative Thoughts

A way to uncover negative thoughts is to keep a *Thought Log*. Remember: your thinking affects your feelings, which in turn affect your behavior. Therefore, examining your negative thoughts is extremely important to the healing process.

A simple way to organize your *Thought Log* is to document the negative thoughts as they pertain to a specific situation. For example, let's examine a common situation – going to a social-get-together. After dinner your favorite seven-layer chocolate cake is served for dessert! Sadly, you have identified the chocolate cake as a "bad" food and therefore it is forbidden. This "bad" connotation sends negative and distorted, even irrational, thinking into play. The thoughts may go something like this, "I can't eat that, it's too fattening! If I eat that, I'll gain ten pounds and become huge. If I become fat, people won't like me, think I'm disgusting, and won't want to be around me. If I am fat and disgusting nobody will love me." All of this negative and distorted thinking was generated by the offer of a piece of chocolate cake! To assist in identifying the distorted thoughts, put them into categories. There are eleven classes of distorted thoughts.

Distorted Thought Categories

1. **Black and White Thinking:** We look at behaviors, as well as the world in general, in all-or-nothing terms. (I can't have just one cookie; it's either none or the whole bag.)

2. **Negative Filter:** We allow ourselves to focus only on the negative and filter out the positive. (Someone gave you a compliment and instead of thinking, "How nice," instead you think, "They don't mean it, they are just trying to be nice.")

3. **Over-Generalization:** We perceive one negative incident as a never ending pattern of doom. (Because I got laid off, I'll never be able to maintain another job.)

4. **Emotional Reasoning:** We use our feelings as evidence or justification. (I feel so dumb, thus I must be stupid.)

5. **"Should" Statements:** Using words like 'should,' 'must,' and 'ought to' is a form of self-criticism. (I should be thinner.)

6. **Devaluing Positives to Bargain-Basement Status:** We negate our positive characteristics and accomplishments and even discount compliments we

receive. (Someone says, "I love your new dress." Your response is, "This old thing? It's only a hand-me-down from my sister.")

7. **Mind-Reading:** Without any evidence, we assume that others are responding to us in a negative way. (That guy didn't ask me out because he thinks I'm fat.)

8. **Fortune-Telling:** We automatically predict that things will turn out for the worst. (I'm not going to try out for the position, since I won't get the part anyway.)

9. **Blame and Personalization:** We deny our role in the problem and don't take responsibility for our own actions; or we blame ourselves for the problem when we are not responsible. ("If my husband hadn't made me go to dinner, I would not have binged," OR "Growing up, if I had been nicer to my sister and hadn't fought so much, then my dad would not have left us.")

10. **Minimizing or Magnifying:** we either deny the importance of an issue or make it more exaggerated than it is. ("I can't die from an eating disorder," OR "I gained 2 pounds, I am now a gross pig.")

11. **Labeling:** Instead of labeling the behavior, we label ourselves. (Instead of saying, "I made a mistake," we say, "I'm a loser.")

Aaron Beck, a psychiatrist, developed a method to challenge distorted thoughts that often keep people stuck and miserable. We have provided a derivative of his method to help you change your negative, and often distorted, thoughts. As shown in the example below, first write a detailed description of the situation. Then list the first thought you can remember when presented with the situation. Try and document any thoughts, which came thereafter. If possible, it is helpful to note any emotions that were triggered, either by the situation or the thoughts. Often, more than one feeling will be triggered. Begin to document your distorted thoughts by utilizing the categories above. Use *Thought Log I* (Figure 6.4 below) to help you organize and document your negative thoughts as they relate to a specific situation.

Figure 6.4: Thought Log I

Describe the situation in detail	List all the negative (distorted) thoughts	Categorize the type of distorted thought	List all the feelings experienced
Offered piece of chocolate cake.	I can't eat that it's too fattening! If I eat that I'll gain 10 lbs.!	Magnification; Black-and-white thinking	Anxiety, fear

PART 2: LET'S CHANGE THAT STINKIN' THINKIN'

Now that you have noted some of your negative and distorted thoughts, it's time to create change. Let's transform the distorted thoughts into more rational, realistic ones. There will be no more allowing your thoughts to run away like a freight train. If you can manage your thoughts, you will create more calm and peace in your life by doing so. Let's look at a previous example on how to change a distorted thought into a realistic thought. Remember the example with the chocolate cake? The thoughts began, "I can't eat that, it's too fattening," and, "If I eat that I'll gain ten pounds." These thoughts would be categorized as Magnification and Black-and-White thinking. Usually, a single thought will fall into more than one category. A rational thought to replace the previous statements would go something like, "Eating one piece of chocolate cake will not make me gain ten pounds," and, "Almost anything in moderation is okay." Now it is your turn to try. Take each hazardous thought and create a more rational statement to replace it. Use figure 6.5: *Thought Log II*, as displayed below, as a template to organize your thoughts.

Figure 6.5: Thought Log II

Describe the situation in detail	List all the negative (distorted) thoughts	Categorize the type of distorted thought	Rational response to negative (distorted) thought
Offered piece of chocolate cake.	I can't eat that it's too fattening! If I eat that I'll gain 10 lbs.!	Magnification; Black-and-white thinking	Eating one piece of chocolate cake will not make me gain 10 lbs. Almost anything in moderation is okay.

We have just explored how negative thinking plays a role in creating a poor body image. We have also seen how our negative thoughts produce negative feelings. We often live life in an automatic fashion and are unaware of our feelings, so we have provided you with a list (See Figure 6.6: *Feeling List*, below). By becoming aware of your feelings you can work backwards and find out what thoughts you were thinking that led to those feelings.

Figure 6.6: Feelings List

Negative Feelings

sad	mad	scared
depressed	angry	helpless
guilty	hostile	submissive
ashamed	hurt	confused
lonely	hateful	insecure
bored	raging	rejected
sleepy	critical	anxious
inferior	jealous	bewildered
inadequate	selfish	insignificant
miserable	frustrated	discouraged
stupid	furious	weak
bashful	irritated	foolish
embarrassed	skeptical	

Positive Feelings

peaceful	powerful	joyful
content	important	excited
thoughtful	faithful	sexy
intimate	hopeful	energetic
loving	appreciated	playful
trusting	respected	creative
nurturing	proud	aware
reflective	confident	delightful
relaxed	intelligent	extravagant
responsive	worthwhile	amused
serene	valuable	stimulated
sentimental	satisfied	fascinated
thankful	cheerful	daring

1. At the end of each day, identify 4 feelings you experienced that day and why.

Example: "I felt sad because my friend cancelled our dinner plans for the evening."

"I felt_____because_____."

"I felt_____because_____."

"I felt_____because_____."

"I felt_____because_____."

Negative feelings can intensify you inner-critic or eating disorder voice. Often the more negative emotions you have in a day, the more likely you are to be dissatisfied with your body. Women often say they "feel fat," although 'fat' is technically not an emotion. The 'fatter' one feels, the more likely one is to engage in disordered eating or eating disorder behavior. Women with anorexia are likely to restrict more, bulimics are likely to binge/purge with more frequency, and compulsive overeaters will stuff their feelings down with additional food.

When a person habitually, emotionally eats versus eating to satisfy their physical hunger, they begin to lose the ability to feed their body appropriately. As you progress in identifying your feelings, you will be less likely to confuse emotional eating and physical hunger. When you are unaware of your feelings, you are more apt to eat unconsciously. In the next section, we explore the difference between physical and emotional hunger.

PHYSICAL HUNGER VS. EMOTIONAL HUNGER

Sometimes distinguishing between physical and emotional hunger can be tricky. Since many of us are cut off from our bodies, we are not alert to the signs of true physical hunger. Emotional eating is common to many of us and often has its roots in early childhood. We become so accustomed to eating, instead of feeling, that our intake is automatic. Some eat compulsively and never actually feel hungry. All of these factors lead to confusion over whether we are actually hungry or emotionally hungry. Ask yourself, "Do I eat because I am hungry or because I want to feed my emotions (bored, sad, lonely, angry, etc.)?" You will probably find that your hunger depends on the time, the meal, and the circumstance. Most people eat breakfast because they are hungry. They have gone several hours since their last meal need to 'refill' their stomachs back up, so to speak. In contrast, people who have eaten three solid meals and have sat at a desk all day do not need to eat all night long in front of the television. It is very unlikely that they are physically hungry; most likely they are either bored, had a rough day and trying to soothe themselves, or are angry and trying to stifle the anger down. Below are lists to clarify the differences between physical and emotional hunger characteristics.

PHYSICAL HUNGER
(INTERNAL MESSAGE)

- Growling stomach
- Desire for a balanced meal
- Slight headache
- Shaky feeling
- Difficulty concentrating
- Low energy level
- Extended time between meals
- Light-headedness

Once you have fed your body, these symptoms are relieved or greatly reduced.

EMOTIONAL HUNGER
(OFTEN A RESPONSE TO AN EXTERNAL SITUATION)

- Intense cravings for specific foods, often high in sugar and/or fat
- No feeling of satisfaction, despite the quantity or what was eaten
- Response to an external trigger (i.e., argument with a significant person, an upsetting phone call, a grade less than perfect on an exam, etc.)
- Feeling a need to hide in order to eat, relating to a feeling of shame about this behavior

The time of day a person eats is often a factor. For example, for many people the evening is a time when they tend to overeat or engage in other unhealthy eating behaviors. By reviewing the "Food" column in your *Physical Hunger vs. Emotional Hunger Table*, you can often tell if you are eating for physical or emotional reasons. If your food is a doughnut at 2:00pm, after you have eaten a big lunch at 1:00 p.m., you are not likely to be feeding physical hunger. The "Amount," and "Degree of Hunger" columns, you can gauge if maybe you should be eating earlier. For example, if you notice that you eat a big lunch at 1:30 p.m. and your degree of hunger is really high, you may need to make an adjustment to having a mid-morning snack or begin eating lunch earlier. In the "Degree of Hunger" column, rate your hunger on a scale of 1 to 5 (1 meaning you are full, 3 meaning you are somewhat hungry, and 5 meaning you are ravenous). At first it may be difficult to gauge your hunger, but by referring to the table you can begin to distinguish between emotional and physical hunger. It is important to avoid waiting to eat until you are ravenous, because by then you will be out of control. On the opposite end, you want to avoid eating when you are full, as that is more likely to be emotional eating. Eating when you are moderately hungry will work out the best.

The last column is the "Emotional Trigger" column (Chapter Nine, *Preventing Relapse* explains in detail what an emotional trigger is and you may want to scan this explanation if you need additional information). In the "Emotional Trigger" column, identify what triggered you to eat. Are there certain situations, people, time(s) of the day, places, or habits, that lead you to eat? Often we have developed what is known as paired-eating. We go to the movies and we want popcorn. It has nothing to do with hunger, but has everything to do with the fact that we are ingrained with the idea of eating popcorn at the movies. We pair certain activities with certain foods, such as peanuts at a ball game. By identifying the paired eating, you can break the pattern. It might feel strange at first, but soon you will be able to go to the movies and be popcorn free!

In the table below record everything you eat, when you eat it, how much you eat, and why. It is important that you keep this record to see if you are eating because you are physically hungry or because you are emotionally hungry.

Figure 6.7: Physical Hunger vs. Emotional Hunger Table

Time	Food	Amount	Degree of Hunger	Emotional Trigger

As you identify your triggers, you will be able to eat more naturally out of physical hunger.

Now that you have completed the *Physical Hunger vs. Emotional Hunger Table*, you are better able to identify the trigger that lead to emotional eating. With this knowledge, you will be able to eat more naturally out of physical hunger. Also, you will need to utilize replacement and nurturing activities. Examples of replacement activities include physically distancing yourself from the food (away from the kitchen), brushing your teeth, chewing gum, or calling a friend. For a list of *Nurturing Activities* refer to Chapter 7.

We have discussed at length issues related to the body and the mind, but have yet to incorporate much about our spirit, which is the supportive foundation of total healing. Many of us who experience emotional hunger are disconnected from our spirit. On the surface our cravings are for food, but at a deeper level we desire spiritual fulfillment. By reconnecting with our spirit we feed ourselves on all levels, thereby not having to stuff ourselves with food. In order for us to create permanent change and a positive body image, we need to nurture and give significant attention to our spirit. The following section addresses this very important element within us all.

HEALING OF THE SPIRIT

Meditation, prayer, reflection, and quiet time are all very relaxing and wonderful tools in healing our body image. Often our body can become separated from our spirit when we have a poor body image, so it is necessary to look at spiritual healing as a part of the total healing process. The body, mind, and spirit, work as one. If one part is damaged it affects the others; therefore, it is necessary to look holistically at healing. Not only do we need to feed our body, but our mind and spirit as well. We know to feed our body we must eat right and to feed our mind we must be mentally active, study, learn, and think positive and uplifting thoughts. But how do we feed our spirit? Many of us do this each week at our church, bible-study groups, or temple, but how do we uplift and feed the spirit daily? The answer is to practice stopping "mind chatter." This exercise is essential for us to communicate with our spirit more clearly. Try this next exercise to help clear your mind and begin feeding your spirit.

THE UPPER ROOM

Read the "Upper Room" exercise in its entirety; then reread it a few more times in order to familiarize yourself with it. When you're done with that, try it for yourself. Before you begin the exercise, start by allowing your body to relax. The purpose of this exercise is to enable you to feel charged with positive energy; this is the food for your spirit. Often people feel drained and depleted, with voids that need to be filled. In order to heal our body image issues, we need to feel complete. This exercise helps in that endeavor.

Sit in a comfortable position in a chair. Uncross your arms and legs, place both feet on the floor, and have your hands in your lap. When you feel comfortable and situated, close your eyes. Now take a deep, slow breath, allowing your breath to expand your abdominal region. Hold your breath for three seconds and slowly exhale. Repeat this breathing sequence until you begin to feel relaxed.

Now that your body and mind are feeling relaxed, focus on a spot six inches above your head. This is called the Upper Room. Experience the energy here, which appears as a crystal white source of light. This light expands into a three-inch star. Continue to focus on your breathing, making sure you are taking deep, relaxed breaths. Now refocus on the Upper Room. Experience the Upper Room filling up and nurturing you with love, support, courage, and wisdom of the Divine. Experience and notice the change as the Upper Room fills up.

Now, shower yourself with the light of the nurturing gifts of love, support, courage, and wisdom. You are filled with goodness in, around, and through you. Feel the shower cleanse away any blocks and obstacles to healing your body image. Let the shower pour out through the bottoms of your feet and into the earth. Now pause.

Now, close off the bottoms of your feet so you can fill back up with these gifts. Fill yourself until you are overflowing. Once you experience the overflow, turn off the downpour and focus back on the Upper Room. Take your time. When you feel comfortable, open your eyes. Know that whenever you need to fill yourself up with these positive gifts, the Upper Room is always open. It is essential that you take only a few minutes of quiet time for yourself to engage in this exercise. The "Upper Room" exercise is based on Actualism. Actualism is a training exercise in meditation and other techniques that opens an individual to their inner source of love, wisdom, and creative expression.

In this exercise, you learned a technique that helps you to experience the essence of the Spirit; a peaceful, loving, radiating presence. We are not talking about religion, which is an individual choice and can also further nurture the Spirit, through fellowship activities and reading. However, essentially all the world's religions and spiritual belief systems have at their core an essence of the Divine. To be able to attune yourself to God or Spirit, that is the way to nurture and feed your spirit. By asking God for the strength and courage to heal, we have added a whole new and very powerful dimension and resource to our healing attempts. Since healing from eating and body image issues is so over-whelming, it is often necessary to turn outside ourselves for help, guidance, and hope. God hears prayers and answers them. Make time to pray, meditate, or talk to God – whatever works best for you. Allow God to be your healing companion. We cannot do it alone. Know God is there for you to help you on your healing journey.

RELEASING YOUR BODY OF NEGATIVITY

Our bodies have been the storehouse for much negativity. We want to help you rid yourself of negativity and fill back up with the positive. To assist you in this process, we have designed a sort of "spring cleaning" visualization exercise. It may be helpful to read through this exercise a few times to get the process clear in your mind, before you embark on the activity. It is important to have your body and mind in a relaxed state during this exercise, so spend a few moments getting yourself centered.

Sit in a comfortable chair or lie down without crossing your arms and legs. Close your eyes and begin to focus on your breathing... Take in very slow and deep breaths... As you inhale, feel your lungs filling to their capacity with oxygen... Picture the oxygen flowing through your body and blood stream, creating a heightened sense of relaxation... As you exhale, let any tension or stress in your body be released through your fingertips and toes... Again, take in a deep breath and exhale slowly... Continue to breathe in this fashion throughout the remainder of the exercise.

VISUALIZATION PART I: SPRING CLEANING

Now it's time to do some spring cleaning of negativity just as you would clean out your closet of clothes you no longer care for or wear. Visualize yourself getting a large plastic bag, the big trash-can type... You will stuff this bag with all the negative thoughts and/or feelings that arise during the exercise... This trash bag is going to be the holding container of the negativity you are going to release from your body... Have a few extra trash bags close by in case the one you are holding gets filled up.

With your eyes closed, spend some time scanning your entire body... Go slowly, going over each and every body part, starting with your toes and feet... Pay close attention to the negative thoughts and/or feelings that pop up as you address each body part... As the negative thought or feeling enters into your awareness, put it into the trash bag... Just as you clean out your closet of unwanted clothes, you clean out your body of unwanted thoughts and feelings... Good. Keep scanning your body; moving to the next area ...your calves... your knees... and your thighs (spend a few moments here since many people have a slew of negativity attached to their thighs)... Now move to your genitals and buttocks... Really take your time... The areas that are the most difficult are the areas we tend to rush through. Continue slowly, progressing upward to your stomach... back... breasts... shoulders... arms... hands... and fingertips... Now focus on your neck... face... and hair... You did it! You have now captured all the negativity that was taking up residence in your body and have put it in the trash bag... Take a few moments to make a list of the contents in your trash bag. List all the negative thoughts and/or feelings in the space provided.

MY TRASH BAG

_____

_____

_____

_____

_____

_____

_____

_____

_____

_____

_____

_____

_____

_____

_____

_____

_____

_____

_____

_____

_____

VISUALIZATION PART II: RECYCLING

Step two in this activity is brief. It is important to once again begin with your body and mind in a relaxed state. So let's start by sitting in a comfortable chair or lying down (without crossing your arms and legs). Close your eyes and begin to focus on your breathing... Take in very slow, deep breaths. As you inhale, feel your lungs filling to their capacity with oxygen. Picture the oxygen flowing through your body and blood stream, creating a heightened sense of relaxation. As you exhale let any tension or stress in your body be released through your fingertips and toes... Again, take in a deep breath and exhale slowly... Continue to breathe in this fashion throughout the remainder of the exercise.

Now see yourself standing in front of your bundled-up trash bags... Pick up your trash bags and load them into your car... You will now get into your car, turn the ignition key, and begin driving to the nearest recycling bin... As you drive, you feel the release and sense of impending freedom as you realize you are fully ridding yourself of this negativity you have been harboring for so many years... You are now pulling into the parking lot and can see the recycling center... Drive to the recycling center and park your car... Your car is now parked and you are exiting your car, going around to the back seat or trunk (wherever you stored your trash bags)... See yourself unloading the bags and handing them to the workers who run the recycling center... Pay attention to the relief and releasing effect this has... The workers take the trash bags from you... This is a very special recycling center, for they know how to recycle negativity and turn it into positive and useful energy... The workers then redistribute this energy to work in a positive way. Great! You have now completed Parts I and II of this activity. Now that you have rid yourself of all this negativity, it is time to fill up that empty space with positive thoughts, feelings, and energy.

VISUALIZATION PART III: LET'S GO SHOPPING

In the next visualization exercise, you can experience filling back up with the positive. Imagine a store filled with beautiful things: objects radiating with happiness and serenity. If we look at the analogy of cleaning out the old and unwanted clothes, what do we typically do with that extra newfound space? Buy more clothes, of course! If shopping has been an out of balance and addictive behavior you have struggled with, you may find the following exercise even more pertinent to your healing. Instead of focusing on accumulating things, you will be focusing on accumulating affirmation and praise. So, once again let's begin by sitting in a comfortable chair or lying down, without crossing your arms and legs... Close your eyes and begin to focus on your breathing... Take in very slow and deep breaths... As you inhale, feel your lungs filling to their capacity with oxygen... Picture the oxygen flowing through your body and blood stream, creating a heightened sense of relaxation. As you exhale, let any tension or stress in your body be released through your fingertips and toes... Again, take in a deep breath and exhale slowly... Continue to breathe in this fashion throughout the remainder of the exercise.

See yourself get into a car and begin to drive to your favorite store, mall, or boutique... You have now parked your car and are entering your favorite store for your shopping excursion. However, it looks quite different than it did before. It is a different type of store. You will be the only shopper, so you can take as much time as you need to "try things on" and not be bothered by other shoppers or sales people. The store is filled with warm feelings and positive energy, it is as though there is an inviting pink haze all about the store that feels very warm, loving, and inviting... You are now in the store and pushing a large shopping cart down the aisle. Allow the pink haze to shower over you, creating a heightened sense of inner peace... As you walk down the aisles, you notice that the items that are hanging on the racks and folded on the shelves are not clothes but words of praise, encouragement, and love... Begin to place these "garments" of love, praise, and encouragement in your shopping cart... Really take your time... You are going to continue to shop until your cart is overflowing... Pay attention to the positive thoughts and feelings that are arising as you place the various "garments" into your cart... You are doing great! Now go over to the full-length mirror that is on one of the sidewalls of the store... It is time to "put on" these positive phrases of love, praise, and encouragement... Slowly take one out of your basket, and put it on – "You are wonderful!" Experience the joy of absorbing the praise... Do not take this garment off; you will continue to add layers... Now put on the next one, "I am loved by many." Repeat this same process until your shopping cart is empty... You are now filled up with and totally surrounded by positive energy through the various words of praise, love, and encouragement... Take a few minutes to document the "new garments" you purchased on your shopping adventure.

MY SHOPPING ADVENTURE

_____
_____
_____
_____
_____
_____
_____
_____
_____
_____
_____
_____
_____
_____
_____
_____
_____
_____
_____
_____
_____
_____
_____
_____
_____
_____
_____
_____
_____
_____
_____

Continue to shower yourself with the new gifts you purchased on your shopping excursion.

Chapter Seven

❦

The Physical Healing Triad

The *Physical Healing Triad* encompasses three components: healthy eating, body movement, and nurturing activities (See Figure 7.1, *Physical Healing Triad*, below). In order to recover from a negative body image and heal your relationship with food, all three components need to be addressed. Healthy eating includes making nutritious food choices, maintaining a good relationship with food, the absence of fat phobia, learning to listen to your hunger, and responding to the feedback your body gives you. The body constantly monitors itself and gives you all kinds of useful, health related information.

Figure 7.1: The Physical Healing Triad

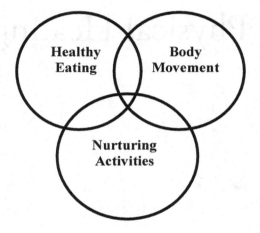

Body movement includes any kind of physical movement. This can be in the form of a regular workout at the gym or fun activities; such as bike riding with people you enjoy, taking a nature walk, or doing some sort of stretches or yoga. The body is designed to move. Before the age of machines, people were on the move much of the day. The body likes to work! A word of caution here: exercise addiction, exercising to the extreme with little food intake and too little rest, is NOT a healthy activity. Make sure you start slowly and don't overdo it. Also, don't forget to begin physical activity with some sort of stretching exercise. If you have a medical condition or have not exercised regularly in some time, you should consult a physician before getting started. You want to strive for a balance of physical exertion and relaxation.

Nurturing activities are very healing. They help us recharge our batteries and rejuvenate ourselves mentally and physically. Taking a bubble bath, listening to soothing music, going to bed early, reading a novel, and lighting scented candles (aromatherapy) are all marvelous nurturing activities (See a complete list of *Nurturing Activities,* later in this chapter). Healthy eating and body movement also fall under this category. In order for the body to stay healthy, it needs to be fed properly, moved (See *Body Movement Exercise,* later in this chapter, for a stretching activity), and be nurtured.

Even though we might constantly strive for perfect health, the truth is there is no such thing. Everyone gets sick, even those who eat right, exercise, meditate, and do all the right things. If they didn't, there would be no need for the healing arts. Perfect health is a wonderful goal and to strive for it is healthy and wise; however, we must realize that sometimes getting sick is a part of life. The body needs downtime. Since many of us do not give the body adequate rest, the body tends to make us sick so we will finally sleep! Balancing the needs of our body is the best way to ensure total health.

ATTRIBUTES OF GOOD HEALTH

- High energy
- Normal laboratory results (blood panel, EKG, etc.)
- A feeling of wholeness and wellness
- Resistance to disease
- Stamina
- Optimism

A person who loves his or her body takes the time and energy necessary to keep it healthy. To maintain good health one needs to make long term changes in ones lifestyle, incorporating healthy eating, body movement, and nurturing activities. The next section focuses on healthy eating.

Healthy Eating

Along with the quest for "perfect" health is the quest for "perfect" eating, but healthy eating is NOT perfect eating. People often get trapped in all-or-nothing thinking about food. They believe that unless they eat freshly grown, organic, unprocessed food at each meal, they have completely failed. While eating such food is healthy, and even an admirable goal, it's just not going to happen for most of us. Does that mean we should abandon our goals for healthy eating? Absolutely not!

People who value health and fitness are interested in feeding their body optimally – a desirable trait. However, some people erroneously believe that "perfect eating" leads to a "perfect body." On the surface this may appear logical, but if you go a little deeper, you can see that this is a trap because eating right does not give you a fantasy body. For example, eating right does not change bone structure, your height, the color of your eyes, etc.

Eating is multidimensional. We eat for any number of reasons: our health, to socialize, for pleasure, because someone offers food to us, because it's time to eat, because there is an opportunity to eat our favorite food, and so on.

Someone with either a poor relationship with food or a negative body image feels that these reasons are wrong or not acceptable to him or her. In fact, what does become acceptable to that person grows smaller and smaller over time, as he or she begins to restrict what is considered safe or appropriate foods. If that trait continues, it leads to full-blown anorexia, and if it still persists, it leads to death. Why? Because at some point there is no "perfect" food, and thus the anorexic does not eat! This behavior is extreme, of course, but it does happen. To avoid constantly feeling like a failure, the key is to know that there is no absolute, perfect diet. However, there are attributes of healthy eating, which are encompassed in the following list.

Attributes of Healthy Eating:

- Choose foods that contain healthy fats like fish, avocado, nuts, seeds, olive oil, flax seed oil, etc.
- Eat a variety of foods

- Include fresh local seasonal produce
- Eat high fiber plant foods
- Choose nutrient-rich foods instead of empty calories (junk food)
- Eat in moderation
- When possible buy unprocessed, unrefined, organic foods
- Keep salt and sugar to a minimum
- Eat a balance of lean protein, healthy fats and low glycemic index carbohydrates
- Enjoy eating!

It is important to try to match your diet (daily food intake) with one that works best for you. Due to biochemical individuality, the diet that is ideal for one person may not be adequate for the next person; however, everyone can benefit from eating vegetables. They provide a wide variety of fiber, vitamins, minerals, and phytochemicals. These compounds keep us healthy and prevent unwanted degenerative diseases. The average American eats less than three servings per day. For optimum health, the recommendation is a minimum of 5 servings per day!

The next component that everyone can agree on is protein. Protein is necessary for numerous life giving processes in the body. Lean proteins include white breast of chicken and turkey. Lean cuts of beef and pork such as flank steak and pork tenderloin are also good sources of protein. The content of fat widely varies in fish, but the omega 3 fat in fish is advantageous to your health. Tofu is a vegetarian source of protein.

Views on fat have changed over the last several years. There are heart-healthy cultures that eat low-fat, such as the Chinese, and heart-healthy cultures that eat high-fat, such as the Eskimos. Fat is necessary for vision, brain development, cell membrane structure, etc. Avoid trans fat, which are found in fried and packaged foods. Look for healthy sources of fat found in fish, nuts, seeds, avocado, olive oil and flax seed oil.

Carbohydrates are the most controversial of the three energy nutrients. Looking at early humans, we find they ate no refined carbohydrates. They subsisted on lean game and green vegetables with the occasional fruit in season, nuts, and honey.

Some people are gluten sensitive, and they must avoid all gluten containing foods to remain healthy. Gluten is found in some grains. Diabetics must carefully select their carbohydrates to control their blood sugar. Truthfully, nobody needs to be eating processed carbohydrates and sugar. They affect the blood sugar, which puts a burden on the body. High fructose corn syrup, found in sodas, is especially damaging to our health. The current recommendation is to eat carbohydrates that are low on the glycemic index. These do not raise blood sugar to the extent that the high glycemic index carbohydrates do. There are several books available with the glycemic index of foods as well as lists on the Internet.

A simple way to evaluate what diet works best for you is to keep a food record. How do you feel after you eat certain foods? Are there times of the day you are more or less hungry? Do you need a higher protein diet or is a balance of carbohydrate, fat, and protein right for you? Use the *Food Record* provided to track your eating so you can begin to understand what plan works best for you. To customize a diet that is suited to your biochemical individuality, consult a knowledgeable nutrition professional.

The *Food Record* (Figure 7.2, below) will give you feedback on how your body likes the diet you have chosen for it. For example, some people eat a very high carbohydrate diet and feel better eating a big lunch. Others need a big, high protein breakfast. Let your body and your *Food Record* be your guide!

Figure 7.2: Food Record

Time	Food	Amount	Feelings

Take a moment to examine your *Food Record*, and then answer the following questions to provide more clarity about your current diet.

1. How do I feel on this diet?

_____

_____

_____

_____
_____
_____

2. Did I eat several servings of vegetables?

_____
_____

3. Did I eat high quality carbohydrates? If yes, what were they?

_____
_____
_____
_____
_____

4. Did I eat healthy fats? If yes, what were they?

_____
_____
_____
_____
_____

5. Did I have enough protein?

_____
_____

6. List the various types of protein you ate?

_____
_____
_____
_____
_____

7. Based on the information you gathered, identify 3 dietary changes you need to make for optimum health.

Dietary Change #1:

_____

_____

Dietary Change #2:

_____

_____

Dietary Change #3:

_____

_____

At the end of the week, review how you feel to see if there are any other changes that need to be made.

BODY MOVEMENT

Our bodies are designed to be in motion. As anyone with a sedentary job knows, a people who sit all day long get back or neck aches, their shoulders roll forward, and they feel stiff. Body movement is essential for good health. People often say, "I know I need to exercise," but in the end, they don't. Clearly, these people either dislike exercise or feel they can't fit it into their busy schedule. Why not start doing a fun physical activity on a regular basis? Such activities can include riding a bike with your kids, pushing your baby in his or her stroller, or taking your dog for a walk. Don't call it exercise, call it playtime! Just make the time to move your body. Once that happens, if you so desire, you can then graduate into something more structured. The point is, don't turn yourself off with the word "exercise." If making exercise fun does not get you to commit to regular physical activity, then a personal trainer may be needed. Finding a way to add exercise to your routine is essential to maintaining a healthy body.

At the other extreme are people who drive themselves into the ground, trying to achieve the perfect body. As we all know, the 'perfect' body is a trap since everyone is unique. The body cannot be transformed (without surgery) into something it is not. People who obsess about their bodies have little time for anything else — they are either exercising, thinking about exercising, or feeling guilty because they haven't been exercising. Once again, somewhere in the middle lies the balance. Regular body movement, coupled with a balanced healthy diet, constitutes health.

Yoga is a great noncompetitive technique to get back in touch with your body, whether you are a couch potato or are exercising your body into the ground. Yoga is an ancient system of exercise that works the entire body, inside and out. There are many different types of yoga, as well as different levels from beginning to advanced. Don't be fooled into thinking that yoga is too easy for you; some postures are very difficult. We recommend a beginning hatha yoga class for getting in touch with your body. There is nothing quite like stretching out your entire body for a deep sense of relaxation.

In her article, "Healing Body Image with Yoga," Gretchen Newmark states, "For many people the body and mind are at war. Yoga makes peace in this conflict by de-emphasizing outward appearance." The focus in yoga is to gradually progress to a state where your body is strong and limber enough to hold a pose. Students of yoga are not focused outwardly. They are completely absorbed in the feedback their body is giving them about its ability to achieve a certain posture. And in our sedentary world, the feedback may not always be pleasant. Anyone who has tried to stretch out a tight muscle knows it can only move as the body allows it to. The body gives loud and precise feedback. If you could hear your body clearly on a daily basis, you would learn to take better care of it. Yoga initiates communication with the body.

Try this next exercise, as part of the body movement component of the physical healing triad, and feel the difference it makes in your body. As we learn to listen and respond to our body, we learn to appreciate it and thus, can learn to love and heal our body image. As you try this exercise, approach it with a positive attitude and allow yourself to relax as you *slowly* stretch your muscles. Enjoy!

BODY MOVEMENT EXERCISE

Find yourself a comfortable chair. Keep your arms and legs uncrossed throughout the exercise. Place both of your feet flat on the floor, and sit up straight (though not rigid). Stretching should be gentle and never painful. During this exercise, breathe slowly and deeply, allowing your lungs to fill to capacity. The more oxygen you take in, the more relaxed your body will feel. Begin by stretching your neck, progressing until you have completed all muscle groups.

1. Neck Rolls

Begin by slowly, not forcefully, rotating your head down so your chin touches your chest. Now, roll your neck to the right so your right ear is near your right shoulder. Next, slowly rotate your head backwards, slightly dropping your jaw open as you tilt your head back. Rotate your neck to the left and then back to the center. Repeat this to the right one more time and then twice to the left.

2. Shoulder Shrug

Lift your shoulders up to your ears. Tighten your arms all the way down and clench your fists. Hold that position with your muscles tense for 5 seconds, and then fully release the tension. Repeat.

3. Arm Lift

Raise your right arm straight up in the air. Really stretch your arm - reach toward the ceiling - stretching your whole right side. Now relax. Repeat. Relax. Now stretch the left side in the same fashion.

4. Shoulder Pull

Lift your right arm straight out in front of you. With your left hand, grab your right upper arm and stretch it across your upper body. Hold. Take a deep breath, and on the exhale deepen the stretch. Relax and repeat with your right arm. Now repeat twice with your left arm.

5. Eye Roll

Work your eye muscles by focusing on the face of an imaginary clock. Start by focusing straight up at the 12 o'clock position (keeping head facing straight ahead) rotating to the right to 1:00, 2:00, and 3:00, continuing on to 12 o'clock. When you get back up to 12 o'clock, rotate in the opposite direction.

6. Palming

Vigorously rub your palms together for five seconds. When your palms become hot, place them over your closed eyes. Feel the relaxing sensation from the warmth.

7. Leg Stretch

Lift your right foot straight in front of you, tensing the muscle all the way up your leg. Hold. Now release and allow your leg to drop to the floor. Repeat. Now repeat twice, using your left leg.

8. Tighten Buttocks

Squeeze your buttocks together very tightly. Hold. Release. Repeat.

Make a commitment to practice this stretching exercise a minimum of three times per week, as part of the body movement component of the physical healing triad. On a scale of 1 to 10 (1=extreme muscle tension, 10=full body relaxation) write down how relaxed you are both before and after the stretching exercise.

	Before: Relaxation Rate (1-10)	After: Relaxation Rate (1-10)
Body Movement Exercise #1		
Body Movement Exercise #2		
Body Movement Exercise #3		

NURTURING ACTIVITIES

The third component of the *Physical Healing Triad* is nurturing activities. Why do we treat ourselves so poorly? We would never think of treating an animal the harsh way we treat ourselves. Our time on this earth is short and precious, so it is high time we allow ourselves to experience joy instead of pain. Learning to love you sounds so easy, and yet for many people it is extremely difficult. Why is it so difficult? There is no simple answer to this question. However, a general answer is that somewhere along the way, you either heard from someone that you were not worthy of love, or through events you experienced (such as trauma or neglect) you came to believe it. When you have an underlying belief that you are not worthy of love or happiness, it is difficult to treat yourself with loving and kind behavior. To create positive change it is important to first "act" in a loving manner toward yourself, then eventually the belief will follow. If you keep yourself grounded in negative beliefs and thoughts, then you stay there. If you keep yourself grounded in positive thoughts, you will experience life more positively.

Another concept that is helpful to remember is, "What you focus upon, you will get more of." Therefore, if you choose to stay focused on the negative, rather than dissipating, the negative tends to become bigger and more overwhelming. For example, what do you think of when you go on a diet? Food! Of course, this will eventually lead to more eating. Whatever we continue to think about will manifest it. If we think nobody will ever like us, then we become unlikable. Conversely, if we believe we are a winner we become one. We are all unique and special creations of God, and we all deserve to experience joy in our lives and be happy. Let's begin to treat ourselves with love, kindness, and nurturance; and leave the self-destructive behavior and thinking behind.

By diligently practicing positive thinking, we begin to treat ourselves better. We begin to nurture ourselves. The ways in which we seek nurturing may be unique to each and every one of us, but every human being seeks it. During the healing process, the concept of self-nurturing is essential in creating a positive body image because a woman who cares about herself takes loving care of her body.

Often we look to others – a spouse, a friend, a family member, a co-worker, etc. – to nurture us. To be nurtured by another is a wonderful experience. However, people can also set themselves up for a major disappointment when continually looking to others to nurture them. This is where the concept of "self-nurturing" comes into play. Let's turn the focus back onto ourselves, in order to nurture and love ourselves, instead of allowing others to be the primary source of nurturing. Prayer is a powerful way to nurture our soul and assist us in taking good care of ourselves. God can and will move you in the right direction if you allow Him to. We must assume the responsibility for nurturing ourselves and getting our needs met.

First of all, it is unrealistic of us to expect others to be capable of meeting all our needs; and second, to always be available to nurture us. These expectations

If you keep yourself grounded in positive thoughts, you will experience life more positively.

By honoring the commitment to self-nurture you are treating yourself with love and respect.

can lead to a great deal of disappointment and are unfair to the other person. The good news is, we are always available to ourselves (for the most part) and can fill ourselves up with nurturing and love. You may be asking yourself, "But how do I do this?" Start by treating yourself in a loving and kind way. Stop the negative self-talk and begin to engage in fun and nurturing activities.

Examine the following list *of Nurturing Activities* in Figure 7.3.

Figure 7.3: Nurturing Activities

Self-nurturing: engaging in healthy activities that promote self-care.

Go for a walk	Listen to your favorite music
Write a letter to a friend	Sing
Journal	Read a "pleasure" book
Call a friend	Visit a friend
Take time out to draw	Finger paint
Listen to soft music by candle light	Do yoga
Give yourself a foot massage	Take a bubble bath
Listen to a relaxation tape	Dance to favorite music
Give yourself a manicure	Give yourself a pedicure
Drink tea by candlelight	Give yourself a facial
Play with a pet	Take a dog to the park
Go for a walk on the beach	Sit in a jacuzzi
Go for a leisurely bike ride	Go for a drive along the coast
Do crafts	Sit under a tree at the park
Read your list of affirmations	Browse in a bookstore
Take a long, hot shower	Go window shopping
Go to a museum	Go to the movies
Rent your favorite video	Give someone a hug
Sew (needle work, e.g.)	Play on swings, jungle gym
Color in a coloring book	Build a sand castle
Buy yourself flowers	Play a game

Commit to doing three nurturing activities this week and every week.

This week I will nurture myself by:

1._____

2._____

3._____

SELF-NURTURING/EATING BEHAVIOR MATRIX

The following, Figure 7.4: *Self-Nurturing/Eating Behavior Matrix*, will help determine your relationship between self-nurturing and eating behavior. Poor eating habits are often coupled with other issues, especially non-nurturing behaviors and negative body image. A negative relationship with food can interfere with our ability to love, accept, and nurture ourselves. By plotting these important relationships, you can clearly see where you need to focus in the healing process.

Figure 7.4: Self-Nurturing/Eating Behavior Matrix

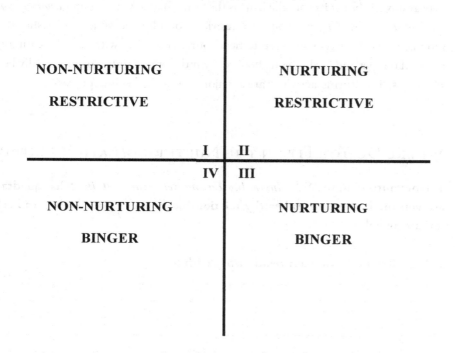

Most women with anorexia nervosa fall into Quadrant I. They diligently restrict their calories and neglect to take care of themselves. They are driving perfectionists who are compelled to do everything right except for self-care. Most women with disordered eating attempt to lead a normal life that includes self-nurturing; however, their weight obsession causes them to unduly restrict calories and be critical about their bodies and thus they belong in quadrant two. Compulsive overeaters, or binge eaters, are usually found in quadrant three. They desire self-nurturing, but unfortunately do so with food. Attempting to nurture with food is really pseudo-nurturing because food cannot fill an emotional void. Most bulimics fall into quadrant four. They have an inner conflict in regards to self-nurturing. They desire to be nurtured, but often feel unworthy. Bulimics, like compulsive overeaters, sometimes use food as a source of pseudo-nurturing. However, the bulimic feels unworthy and guilty for haven eaten, and thus feels compelled to get rid of the food. Of course, healthy women cluster around the center of the matrix. They generally take time to feed themselves properly and balance eating with healthy self-nurturing activities.

Your relationship with food must change.

Depending on the quadrant you find yourself in, the healing strategies may appear to vary, but at its core the issue is the same for everyone. *The relationship with food must change.* Whether you are a restrictor or a binger, your relationship with food is not healthy. As you begin to heal your relationship with food by eating for physical hunger and health, you allow yourself the opportunity to emotionally heal. Healthy self-nurturing activities are a major part of the healing process.

WHERE DO YOU FIT ON THE NURTURING/EATING MATRIX?

1. Plot yourself on the *Self-Nurturing/Eating Behavior Matrix*. What quadrant are you in? Is there an unhealthy relationship between your eating and self-nurturing habits?

2. Describe, in detail, your relationship with food.

_____

_____

_____

_____

_____

_____

_____

_____

_____

_____

It doesn't matter what you weigh or how little you eat. If you don't make the effort to learn to love your body (See Chapter 5, *Choosing a Healthy Body Image*), no matter what you look like, you will stay locked in the prison of self-hate and food phobia. Food is not bad, fat is not bad, and you are not bad. You are a beloved child of God. Healing from disordered eating is a battle. There are many support groups to help you heal, but you must understand that you are more than how your body looks. It is important to follow a regular eating system regardless of how you feel, whether negative or positive. Use your positive affirmations to challenge your negative thinking. Eat regularly scheduled meals until you learn to honor your body and really tune in to it. You can, you must, and you will recover from disordered eating!

NURTURING THE INNER INFANT

As part of the self-nurturing process, we have created a helpful guided imagery for you to utilize as part of your recovery process. Self-nurturing is a skill everyone needs, but is difficult to practice. We are often good at nurturing others, but not so well at nurturing ourselves in a healthy way. This next exercise is designed to access your God-given ability to nurture so that you may transfer this skill to yourself. Read *Nurturing the Inner Infant* a few times thoroughly before doing the guided imagery exercise to become familiar with it.

Sit in a comfortable position in a chair. Uncross your arms and legs, place both feet on the floor, and hands in your lap. When you feel comfortable and situated, close your eyes. Now take a deep, slow belly breath, allowing the breaths to expand your abdominal region... Hold your breath for three seconds and exhale slowly, forcing out all the tension as you exhale... Repeat this breathing sequence until you begin to feel relaxed... Remember, the slow, deep breathing is important during the entire exercise, since an increased level of oxygen helps your body to relax.

Now that you are relaxed, think of a newborn baby... Take the baby in your arms... Notice how you are holding him/her... Are you cradling the baby in your arms while looking into his/her eyes? ... Carrying the baby over your shoulder? ...Are you talking to him/her? ... If so, what things are you saying to the baby? ... Maybe you are gently singing to him/her... Do you notice yourself stroking the baby or rocking the baby? ... Maybe you are feeding the baby... How are you interacting with the baby? ... How are you conveying your feelings of love and acceptance to him/her? ... I want you to hold on to the thoughts and feeling you experienced while nurturing this baby... Again, take a moment to embrace the warmth and love you receive from nurturing this baby and hold it within your heart... When you are ready and comfortable, open your eyes and remember all the necessary details to complete the remainder of this exercise.

1. Describe how you held the baby and the feelings this evoked for you?

_____

_____

_____

_____

_____

_____

2. How did you nurture this baby and demonstrate your love and acceptance to him/her?

_____

_____

_____

_____

_____

_____

3. List 6 things you will do to treat yourself more like a precious infant to give yourself the tender, loving care you deserve.

_____

_____

_____

_____

_____

_____

Commit to these self-care behaviors on a weekly basis.

Chapter Eight

❧

Creating Body-Love

The entire concept of this book is to create body-love. We, Tami and Lisa, want negativity and body-hatred to be a part of your past. You may be saying, "Well, that sounds great, but…" Guess what, there are no "buts" about it. As you read in Chapter Four, you are taking an *active* role in creating change in your life. To create body-love you need to love your body and treat it with the utmost respect and kindness every day. Your body deserves to be treated well. As you become consistent with treating your body in a gentle and loving manner, you will notice a difference in how you feel about yourself. The next exercise is designed to open up the lines of communication between you and your body, which is instrumental in creating body-love.

LEARN TO TALK WITH YOUR BODY

The first question that comes to mind is, "Why do I hate my body so much?" Not only women, but also many men are now acknowledging body-hatred. Instead of addressing our negative feelings, we project them onto the body and store them there. The body then becomes a hated, loathed, and despised object. When the body is objectified in this manner, a split or separation occurs between the self (who you are) and the body.

To heal and recover from a negative body image we must work at reuniting our self and body as well as learn to love our body. Body-hatred begins in the mind (the thought processes), and is followed by negative, destructive behavior. Have you ever caught yourself thinking or saying such body-hatred statements as, "I hate my hips, my buttocks, and my tummy," or, "My breasts aren't big enough!"

Negative and destructive behaviors soon follow these negative thoughts, especially as the negative statements increase in frequency. Have you ever abused your body with drugs, alcohol, destructive eating, or starvation? Have you ever hit yourself, deliberately harmed yourself physically, or put yourself in dangerous and risky situations? All of these behaviors are self-destructive; and neither you nor your body deserves the abuse and destruction you have experienced. Body-hatred can result not only from negative thoughts about our bodies, but also from the experience of any type of abuse: verbal, sexual, physical, or other. People who have been subjected to abuse learn to take out their negative emotions on themselves, even to the point of being self-destructive. The experience of abuse can strip us of self-worth and self-esteem. Body-hatred can also result from growing up in an environment where there was no modeling of self-respect, self-nurturing, self-care, or how to treat our bodies with kindness. Such neglect and abuse often engenders a great deal of anger, which is then projected onto the body as though the body allowed the abuse to happen. If you have experienced any type of abuse and are having difficulty moving past it, counseling from a trained professional may be very helpful.

It is time for you to have a heart-to-heart talk with your body, and for your body to get really honest with you! Your body will tell you how it feels you have treated it. It may seem rather peculiar to have a conversation with your body, but to get reacquainted a dialogue is necessary. Set aside some quiet time for yourself when you will not be distracted or interrupted. Take a moment to close your eyes and scan your body, paying close attention to any thoughts, feelings, and/or images that arise. Now, pick up a pen or pencil and in the space provided write a letter to your body, telling it your comfort level with it and your feelings about it. (Be specific.)

LETTER TO MY BODY

_____

_____

_____

_____

_____

_____

_____

_____

_____

_____

_____

_____

_____

_____

_____

_____

_____

Great job; you did it!!! Take a moment to read your letter aloud. Let yourself experience whatever feelings arise.

1. How did it feel to write this letter?

_____

_____

_____

_____

_____

2. How did it feel when you read the letter aloud?

_____

_____

_____

_____

_____

_____

3. Write a few lines about your experience with this exercise.

_____

_____

_____

_____

_____

_____

Give yourself a big hug and a pat on the back; you deserve it.

THE BODY'S RESPONSE

Now, your body is going to have the opportunity to respond to the letter you wrote to it. It is important for your body to get really honest with you and share how it truly feels about the treatment it has received. Sometimes this exercise can evoke emotions, so make sure you complete this exercise at a moment when you have some quiet, private time. It may be helpful to once again read the letter you wrote to your body before your body writes to you. After you have reread the letter, close your eyes and take a moment to scan your body, paying attention to any thoughts, feelings, and/or images that surface. Pick up your pen or pencil and, in the space provided, have your body write a letter to you about how you've treated or are treating it.

MY BODY'S LETTER TO ME

_____
_____
_____
_____
_____
_____
_____
_____
_____
_____
_____
_____
_____
_____
_____
_____
_____
_____
_____
_____
_____
_____
_____

Take a moment to check in with yourself.

1. How do you feel about writing this letter?

_____
_____
_____
_____
_____
_____
_____

2. What did you learn or discover from this letter?

_____
_____
_____
_____
_____
_____
_____

3. Did your body have important and valuable information to tell you?

_____
_____
_____
_____
_____
_____
_____

4. As you did with the first letter, read this letter aloud to yourself. Allow yourself to experience any feelings that arise as you read the letter. Write a few lines describing your experience with this exercise.

_____
_____
_____
_____
_____
_____
_____

MAKING AMENDS TO MY BODY

It is now time to write a third letter. In this letter, write from the heart. Make amends to your body for the poor treatment it has received as a result of your disordered eating/eating disorder. If you have difficulty getting started, reread the letter your body wrote to you. This is an important part of the healing process. Fight the urge to skip over this exercise; it will be well worth your time!

LETTER OF AMENDS

_____

_____

_____

_____

_____

_____

_____

_____

_____

_____

_____

_____

_____

_____

_____

_____

_____

_____

_____

_____

To make significant change in regard to your body image, changing your thoughts and behavior is important. Ask yourself the following questions and respond to them in the space provided.

1. How are you going to treat your body differently?

_____

_____

_____

_____

_____

_____

2. What loving and nurturing activities are you willing to do this week? (Minimum of three)

a._____

b._____

c._____

3. Write three loving statements to your body.

a._____

b._____

c._____

Whisper "Sweet Somethings" to yourself.

TALK TO YOUR BODY GUIDED IMAGERY

The purpose of this exercise is to help heal the wounds that have been inflicted over the years between you and the various parts of your body you dislike (or maybe even despise).

Sit comfortably in a chair with your feet and arms uncrossed. Close your eyes. Take three slow, deep belly-breaths. Allow yourself to relax. If your mind starts to wander gently refocus on your breathing. Good.

Imagine yourself entering a theater... The lights are low except for the stage, which is illuminated... Walk slowly up the aisle... Stop at the front row and have a seat... See yourself breathing slowly and deeply... Allow the parts of your body you dislike the most, sit next to you... As they take their seats, walk up to the middle of the stage where there is a circle of chairs and sit down... Look down into the first row and ask the first body part to come have a seat beside you...

Scoot your chairs close so you are facing each other... Good.

Begin by introducing yourself to your body part and then have your body part introduce itself to you... Tell your body part that you welcome them here today and appreciate their coming... Admit to your body part that you have hated it for a long time... You wish that it could be changed and be perfect... You are even angry that your body part isn't exactly how you want it to be... Once you have spoken your mind, allow your body part to speak... Let it tell you the depths of the pain it has felt from being unloved... Give your body part time to express the sorrow and anger it is holding in... Allow your body part time to talk to you, without interrupting... When she is done have her go back and sit in the first row.

Now have the next body part come on to the stage and sit across from you... Continue the above dialogue with each body part you dislike to complete this exercise.

Give yourself a big pat on the back this was a tough exercise! Now take a few minutes to write down the primary response each body had in dialoguing with you during this exercise. For further insight on this exercise, answer the process questions. These questions may provide valuable information regarding your healing journey.

Body Part	Primary Response

1. Overall, what did you learn from this exercise?

_____

_____

_____

_____

_____

_____

2. Does continuing to hate/dislike your body wound you? In what ways does it do this?

_____

_____

_____

_____

MAKING AMENDS

1. Does it make sense to continue to hate/dislike your body? Why?

_____

_____

_____

_____

2. Can you see a time when you love and accept your body (even if you are in the process of trying to gain or lose weight or trying out a new look)? Yes or No?

3. What can you do today to establish a better relationship with your body?

_____

_____

_____

_____

_____

Regardless of your body shape, size, or weight, it is time to embrace your body and shower it with the love and kindness it wants and deserves!

POSITIVE BODY TALK

An important part of self-nurturing and learning to love your body is what we call "positive body talk." So much time is spent on criticizing the body that these negative statements become part of your belief system about you. As you begin to love your body, it is important to reunite your self (who you are) with your body. We no longer want our body to be the hated object that, through this hatred, became a separate entity. Just as you had the power to negate and hate your body, creating this separation, you have the power to love and reunite your body and your self. Regardless of your body shape, size, or weight, it is time to embrace your body and shower it with the love and kindness it *wants* and *deserves!*

Love is a powerful emotion and has a tremendous capability to heal. Look to the source of inner love you possess and start treating yourself in this fashion. Treat yourself in the same manner you would treat a significant someone special in your life whom you admire and adore. Love is the special gift you can give yourself and you deserve it!!! You are a special and unique creation of God and you are worthy and deserving of health, happiness, and joy. Take a few moments to complete the following exercise Figure 8.1: *Positive Body Talk.*

Make a commitment to treat yourself and your body with loving-kindness; you are worth it!

Figure 8.1: Positive Body Talk

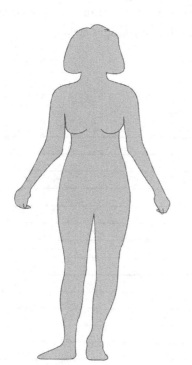

1. In the area above your head, list the characteristics of your spirit.

2. On the face portion of the picture, write three positive statements to help unite your spirit and your body. (e.g. "My body is a beautiful temple that houses my spirit.")

3. Where your heart would be, list at least three ways you can be good to yourself.

Now that you have completed items 1-3 on the *"Positive Body Talk"* exercise, make a commitment to yourself to read over this exercise on a daily basis.

Positive body talk is really about showering your body with kind and loving words and behaviors. Now it's time to create some type of loving tribute to your body.

A LOVING TRIBUTE TO YOUR BODY

As you continue to learn to love your body, it is important to treat it with loving kindness and praise. This exercise leans to the creative side of expression. We want you to write either a poem or a song about your body. There is one stipulation: the song or poem must be written in a positive way so that it affirms your body. Be creative and have fun with it! Really toot your own horn. Lavish your body with kindness; really lay it on thick. If you have trouble doing this, you may want to go through the workbook one more time. Another way is to think of yourself as a young child. It was often easier to praise yourself at a younger age.

MY SONG/POEM

_____

_____

_____

_____

_____

_____

_____

_____

_____

_____

_____

_____

_____

_____

_____

Use the space provided to draw a picture that symbolizes the song or poem you wrote about your body.

Collage: The Transformed Me

It's time to take a look at any transformations that have taken place in your body image. To do this collage, cut out pictures from magazines or books that depict your improved body image, healthy body, new eating habits, and/or general fitness. Resist the temptation to zero in on weight. Instead, focus on the benefits of healthy exercise, nutritious food, high energy, and radiant skin. Look for healthy, active bodies and women who look like they are having fun with appropriate physical activity. If the images in magazines are too thin, as they often are, or looking through the magazines is too much of a trigger for you regarding the unrealistic ideal body, draw your own picture of a healthy body. Also, cut out words, phrases, and scenes that depict the new you. When you finish collecting the images, glue them to the poster board. When you are through, you will have the new you in living color right before your eyes. Congratulations!

1. In creating your collage, did you choose healthy images and positive phrases that support your transformed body image? Write about the images and words you chose for this collage.

_____

_____

_____

_____

_____

_____

_____

_____

a. List the ways in which you transformed your body image. Be specific. What tools and exercises were most helpful for you?

_____

_____

_____

_____

_____

_____

_____

_____

_____

_____

b. If you still feel there is work to be done to meet your body image goal, make a list of activities you can do to continue to create positive change regarding your body image. Remember perfection is not the target, loving your body is.

_____

_____

_____

_____

_____

_____

_____

_____

_____

_____

Congratulations on the progress you have made creating a healthy body image. We know how difficult it is, and how much time and effort you have put into this process. As with any goal, outside pressure can push you off-track. Be prepared for this. If you find yourself becoming critical of your body again, refocus your efforts without feeling guilty or like a failure. It is normal to temporarily lapse, especially because society is so fixated on an unrealistic, and often unhealthy, body-type.

ॐ

Give yourself words of praise and encouragement for the changes you have made!

Chapter Nine

Preventing Relapse

LEADING A BALANCED LIFE

When we feel out of control when we feel wrung out, stressed out, tired and on edge, we tend to gravitate back to old, repetitive behaviors. If those behaviors are destructive, we can get caught up in them all over again. For someone who struggles with poor body image and eating issues, these behaviors can re-emerge during tough times. Though tough times do happen to everyone on occasion, it is important to try to keep balance in your life to prevent slipping back into old, destructive behavior. A balanced life includes many things. We have family, home, work, and other obligations that are necessary, but we need to balance these things with fun-filled play-time (as well as quiet time and relaxation). This way we can feed our Body, Mind, and Spirit.

Throughout the book, *Love Your Body: Change the Way You Feel About the Body You Have,* we have talked about the healing that takes place on interconnecting levels. In the *Physical Healing Triad,* (Chapter Seven) we learned to eat right, exercise, and partake in nurturing activities. In the *Emotional Healing Triad* (Chapter Six), we saw the need to change our thinking, got in touch with our feelings and expressed them in appropriate ways, and partook in nurturing activities. Now it is time to integrate all aspects of healing into our everyday life. This furthers your healing, allows you to lead a balanced life, and helps you prevent relapsing into self-defeating behaviors. See Figure 9.1: *Total Healing Diagram,* to further conceptualize this process.

Figure 9.1: Total Healing Diagram

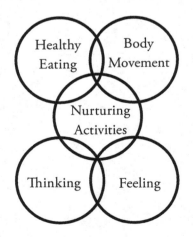

Here we will summarize the "feeding" process for the Body, Mind, and Spirit. The body is fed through food, movement, nurturing activities, positive thinking, and constructive feelings. The brain or mind is fed through mental activity, expansion of knowledge, and proper nutrition; as well as positive thoughts, a stimulating environment, and constructive feelings. The spirit is fed through prayer, meditation, giving, forgiving, and love. It takes discipline to keep focused on the positive. We need to continue to work, using all the techniques we have learned to prevent us from resorting back to the negative. You already know that life has its bumpy moments. Part of success is resetting. When you find yourself veering off course, refrain from self-criticism and simply say to yourself, "I am resetting and am back on course." It is important to get back on track as quickly as possible to prevent backsliding into old destructive habits. Avoid the tendency to overanalyze the situation, which may keep you stuck. After resetting and getting yourself back on course, you can take the time to journal and learn the lessons from the temporary lapse.

Our cultural fantasies make it extremely difficult to avoid lapse and relapse in body image and eating issues. Positive self-talk is essential to counter the "Am I good enough?" chatter that inevitably comes up. Let's look at Figure 9.2: *Progression of Poor Body Image,* to see how the problem begins and advances so we can recognize how to stop it.

Figure 9.2: Progression of Poor Body Image

<u>Problem</u> ⟶ <u>Manifestation</u> ⟶ <u>Action</u> ⟶ <u>Outcome</u>
Weight Phobia   Fear of Fat   Restrictive   Poor Body
    Eating   Image

Initially, the problem is identified as weight phobia. Body size is a seemingly universal condition in our culture today. Women want to be thin, sometimes at all costs. The fear of gaining weight is seen even in our children. Eighty-one percent of all 10-year-old girls are afraid of being fat (Mellin, et. al., 1991). The fear of gaining weight leads to fat phobia. We become terrified of every morsel we put in our mouths. Every bit of food must be scrutinized. The potential for weight gain lurks everywhere. We become paranoid and hypersensitive at every meal. A destructive eating pattern sets in. As the eating pattern becomes more and more restrictive, nutritional deficiencies occur, affecting our thinking and perpetuating a negative pattern. The result is fear of food, obsession with thinness, avoidance of social activities, and low self-esteem, all of which tie right back into and reinforce our poor body image.

To prevent relapse, it is important to remember the genetic variations found within the human structure, to embrace them, and to accept varying weight distribution as normal and beautiful. To review, the three major types of body types are ectomorph, endomorph and mesomorph. Ectomorphs' structures are lean, with small hips and shoulders; long distance runners are ectomorphs. Mesomorphs are muscular, have big and broad shoulders; body builders are mesomorphs. Endomorphs are more rounded; cold-water swimmers are endomorphs. Most people are a combination of two or more types. Each of these shapes is God-given and has unique talents. By embracing each and every shape and size, we prevent the cultural stigma, which leads to body-hatred. By observing people we see the great variety of shapes available in the human form. Instead of thinking critical thoughts about their bodies, or ours, we need to see ourselves and others as unique, loving children of God. By learning to love, accept, and tolerate others, we can learn to love, accept, and tolerate ourselves.

By embracing each and every body shape and size, we prevent the cultural stigma, which leads to body-hatred.

1. For practice, affirm someone else aloud twice per day for the next week.

Example: "I love the way you carry yourself."

Day 1

Affirmation #1_____

Affirmation #2_____

Day 2

Affirmation #1_____

Affirmation #2_____

Day 3

Affirmation #1_____

Affirmation #2_____

Day 4

Affirmation #1_____

Affirmation #2_____

Day 5

Affirmation #1_____

Affirmation #2_____

Day 6

Affirmation #1_____

Affirmation #2_____

Day 7

Affirmation #1_____

Affirmation #2_____

NEGATIVE BELIEFS

We would venture to say that most people, and certainly those who struggle with a poor body image, have many negative beliefs about themselves. These beliefs often begin as thoughts but when rehearsed often enough become a part of our belief system. It is important to identify these beliefs so we can challenge and change them. Much of our negative thinking is automatic, as we discussed in Chapter Six, so we must pay close attention to our thoughts in order to identify the underlying beliefs. A thought has much less significance than a belief, and is therefore a lot easier to let go of. Our beliefs are very solidly entrenched in us and therefore require us to do a great deal of challenging and to be consistent in our efforts to change them. All too often our core beliefs are determined early on, and we assume they are true and a necessary part of ourselves. They are not necessarily true, especially the negative ones.

*We can come to love
ourselves and accept
our bodies just the
way they are.*

We can come to love ourselves and accept our bodies just the way they are. Let's look at an example. Colleen decides she needs to heal her body image and agrees to go to counseling and do her homework; she is committed to working on bettering herself. As part of this process she begins to journal. She has also been instructed to do nurturing activities regularly. As Colleen begins to journal about this a little automatic voice in her head says, "You should be able to do this yourself; this isn't hard. Why are you paying that money for counseling anyway?" She is probably not even aware of what is going on inside her head. As a result of her thoughts, she cancels her appointment. She does not follow through on the nurturing activities or other homework, and she falls back into the trap of hating her body even more.

This is a vicious and unconscious game. To catch yourself, make sure that when you start slipping on your commitments, you immediately stop and ask yourself "What is really going on here?" More often than not, difficult material, feelings, or issues are surfacing, and a great way to get away from them is to stop the process. The sad thing here is that when the process is stopped, healing does not occur. It may even get worse for you because issues have been uncovered so you are more sensitive and vulnerable. We strongly suggest you process through this time of vulnerability. It will get better.

Remember that your inner critic, or eating disorder voice, may re-emerge at any time. Your inner critical voice tends to pop up when you are most vulnerable. *As the potential to relapse increases, the louder the voice gets.* This is the time to use all the tools you have learned to maintain a positive body image.

*Support,
encouragement,
direction, and
accountability are
important and are
a necessary part of
healing.*

Just catching yourself in the act of self-sabotage is not enough. You need to replace the unconscious negative belief with a new belief, one that allows change and growth to take place. In other words, you need to challenge the old negative beliefs that keep you down and stuck! For example, Colleen could have written in her diary a counter to her negative belief that might have gone something like, "Support, encouragement, direction, and accountability are important and are a necessary part of healing, and I get these in counseling."

As you keep your journal over time, you may begin to notice patterns developing. You may find that you use money as an obstacle, time factors, or numerous other excuses for not pursuing your healing efforts. Write in your journal your belief system, and identify the blocks that keep you from progressing. See Figure 9.3: *Belief Journal*, below. Complete the Belief Journal and answer the following questions to summarize your findings.

Figure 9.3: Belief Journal

My Limiting Beliefs	Obstacles	New Belief
This is stupid. I can do this myself. I don't need counseling.	Time Money	I need encouragement, direction and account-ability for healing, and I get this in counseling.

1. What are my four most common beliefs that impede my progress in healing? (If you don't know, you might ask others what is the limiting phrase you frequently say: Or sit in silence and see what comes up for you.)

a._____

b._____

c._____

d._____

2. What are four corresponding challenging beliefs that I can say to help heal my body image?

a._____

b._____

c._____

d._____

EMOTIONAL TRIGGERS

You may be wondering, what is an emotional trigger? It is some type of external stimuli or situation that you respond to internally, often first by thought then by a feeling. Some people, when emotions are triggered, eat to try to comfort, soothe, and nurture themselves, which can lead to a very destructive cycle. For example, it is common for people to turn to food after a stressful day at work. Instead of relieving their stress in healthy ways (e.g., talking to their boss, setting boundaries with co-workers, etc.) they use food as a stress reducer. As part of the healing process, it is important to be able to identify your own emotional triggers so you can respond constructively to your feelings when they do get triggered. And they will!

Remember the *Food Record* in Chapter Seven? This record can give priceless information as to what the emotional triggers are that cause you to eat. Anger, sadness, loneliness, rejection, and boredom are some of the common feelings that people try to soothe or escape from by comforting themselves with food. Go back over your *Food Record* and try to uncover the feelings that trigger you to eat. If you are having difficulty figuring out what you are feeling, look at the *"Feeling List"* in Chapter Six, to assist you in labeling your feelings. It is also helpful to document the type of food you typically reach for in relation to specific feelings. For example, there was a client whom we shall call Mary, who whenever she got angry, would eat her favorite candy bars. The food pattern is not always as clearly defined as it was with Mary, but you can be certain that if you track your food intake with the *Food Record* for any length of time, you will begin to see trends within different food groups, or the avoidance of food groups, related to your emotional triggers.

Take some time to examine your *Food Record*. Make a note as to the situation, the feeling experienced, and the food you chose to eat, and document it in the chart on the following page (See Figure 9.4: *Trigger Chart*, below). Now take some time to fill in the chart. By documenting these details you can be more in the driver's seat than your feelings or disordered eating habits. Remember the goal is to eat for physical hunger, not emotional hunger.

Figure 9.4: Trigger Chart

Situation	Feeling	Food Eaten
Argument with Mom on the phone.	Angry, Anxious, Invalidated	Chocolate Cupcake, ½ bag Potato Chips

HEALTHY WAYS TO HANDLE EMOTIONAL EATING

Now that you have identified and made a list of your emotional triggers, let's discuss more productive ways to handle them than turning to food. The whole destructive cycle of body-hatred often occurs when you seek food as a way to cope with your feelings. Because you have turned to food to try to make yourself feel better, you feel guilty for eating when you weren't really hungry. Then body loathing enters the picture.

The key to growth and change is learning to externalize and express your feelings in healthy ways. This is so very important for one simple reason: your feelings hold a great deal more power and intensity if you keep them inside. There are different ways to externalize or express your feelings. The first would be to talk about your feelings. Find someone you feel safe and comfortable with and tell them what happened (the situation) and what you are feeling. If there is not somebody physically around you to talk to, make a phone call.

There is yet another option open to you for expressing your feelings, and that is journaling. There may not always be someone available to you, either in person or by phone, but you can always find a piece of paper and a pen to journal. (Use toilet paper if you have to!) Some people say they are uncomfortable with journaling because they are afraid somebody is going to stumble across their writings. A good solution to this problem is either to rip up or burn your writings once you have completed them.

Another technique that is helpful when you become emotionally triggered and the refrigerator or cupboards are calling your name is to remove yourself from that environment. Go for a walk around the block, take your dog to the park, or go to a friend's house – anything to get yourself away from the temptation of food. If fast food is a temptation for you, do not bring any money, credit cards, or ATM cards with you when you leave the house. Then try journaling when the food doesn't seem like such a threat.

Learn to externalize and express your feelings.

Sometimes journaling in the form of letter writing is extremely helpful. Say your husband just phoned you and told you that the trip to Hawaii you had been planning for the past six months had just been canceled. You became upset, raised your voice, and he hung up on you. Here you are left with all these emotions and you feel like you are going to explode! This is a prefect time to implement the letter writing type of journaling. Sit down and write him a letter, totally uncensored, with your raw emotions, telling how you feel about this situation. After you have completed the letter, read it aloud as though you were reading it to him, and then rip it up. This may sound like a really silly thing to do, but it is a very useful technique. It allows you to return to your center more quickly and gives you a greater sense of control.

Anxiety is an emotion many individuals experience and struggle with. It is often triggered when we try something new, such as trying to create change in our lives. As part of preventing relapse, we have designed an exercise to combat any anxiety that may surface as you let go of your negative body image to create a more positive, healthy one. Some people experience anxiety in a more extreme form than others – such as panic attacks, which may need medication – and if left untreated can become quite debilitating. Anxiety is an important topic to address because most individuals who struggle with a negative body image experience anxiety about the size and shape of their bodies.

The emotion of anxiety is two-fold, in that it not only creates emotional turmoil, but the body also responds with various physiological symptoms. Here is a list of some of the physiological symptoms of anxiety:

- Increase in heart rate
- Heart palpitations
- Pain, pressure or tightness in the chest
- Restlessness or jumpiness
- Fatigue
- Trembling or shaking
- Muscle tension
- Headaches or pains in the neck or back
- Dizziness or lightheadedness
- Nausea
- Sweating not related to heat
- Diarrhea or other abdominal distress
- Frequent urination
- Irritability
- Hot flashes or chills
- Trouble falling asleep or staying asleep
- Difficulty concentrating or mind going blank
- Shallow breathing

This is not to say that all people who feel anxious will experience all of the above listed physical symptoms, but many people experience a few. Anxiety can manifest itself in different ways for different people. It is very important not to ignore anxiety, but rather to face it and address it head on. This means

Be an active participant n your own healing process.

externalizing the feelings by talking or writing about them, as well as utilizing techniques to relax yourself. Some people who refuse to address their anxiety will end up with physical ailments such as ulcers or colitis. Be an active participant in your own healing process. You are worth it!!!

1. List the physiological symptoms of anxiety you have experienced when feeling anxious. These identified symptoms can be used as a tool to get your attention in recognizing when you are feeling anxious. With this awareness, you can then use one of the relaxation exercises you have learned in this book to help your body relax the *Upper Room (*Chapter 6*)* or *The Body Movement Exercise* (Chapter 7).

_____

_____

_____

_____

_____

_____

_____

Making assumptions or predictions about some future event creates anxiety.

How is the emotion of anxiety created? It's created when an individual starts making assumptions or predictions about some *future* event. This is exciting news! *If one stays grounded in the present moment, anxiety cannot exist;* for some people, however, this is somewhat difficult to do. Look at some examples from your own life. When you have felt anxious, chances are you were ruminating and feeling anxious about some future event (e.g. your chemistry final on Friday, the in-laws coming to visit for a week, your blind date on Saturday). However, people who are habituated to anxiety require many hours of practice to retrain the Mind/Body/Spirit to respond to stress with calm, serenity, and relaxation. Some people are raised in household environments that are filled with chaos and create constant anxiety. A person actually becomes hardwired to expect anxiety. When there is none it feels wrong. If you are one of those people, you may have to work harder to learn to manage your anxiety.

If one stays grounded in the present moment, anxiety cannot exist.

Since anxiety is a reality and an emotion most people have experienced at least once in their lives, let's talk about the ways to manage and minimize anxiety. One of the easiest and most productive techniques you can practice for yourself when you even anticipate feeling anxious is to begin to take very slow, deep breaths to increase the amount of oxygen in the blood stream. When people become anxious their breathing usually becomes more rapid, leading to shallow breaths, which results in a reduction of the level of oxygen in the blood stream, which in turn creates an increase in heart rate and sets off other physiological responses in the body.

Begin to breathe in a slow and very deep breathing pattern. Really try to fill your lungs to their full capacity, and then slowly exhale. As you inhale, allow yourself to feel your heart rate slowing down and your body beginning to relax. As you exhale, feel and visualize any muscle tension or stress in your body exit throughout your extremities (fingertips and toes). Repeat the process until your body has returned to a more relaxed state. This exercise in itself should slow down the physiological response to anxiety and create a feeling of relaxation. You may also wish to repeat the *Upper Room* (Chapter 6), and *Body Movement Exercises* (Chapter 7).

VISUALIZATION ACTIVITY: LET'S WIPE THAT ANXIETY RIGHT OUT OF YOUR LIFE

We would like to guide you through a visualization exercise to rid yourself of your anxiety. It is important to pick a time when you have some privacy and won't be interrupted. Either lie down on the floor or bed or sit comfortably in a chair (legs uncrossed and touching the floor). Close your eyes and begin to take in deep, slow breaths, allowing your body to relax. As you exhale, feel any tension or stress you may have in your body exit through your fingertips and toes. Continue to breathe slowly and deeply throughout the visualization exercise. Good. Your body is feeling more and more relaxed.

Now that you are feeling more relaxed, picture a green chalkboard in front of you, the kind you used to see in your classroom at school... You are in this classroom by yourself and feel serenity here... Let yourself focus on the completely blank chalkboard in front of you ... At the bottom of the chalkboard, you can see several pieces of chalk lying in the tray... The chalkboard has a peaceful and inviting feel to it... See yourself slowly approaching the chalkboard... Again, you are feeling very calm and relaxed... Watch yourself pick up a piece of chalk and just simply hold it in your hand for a few minutes... The chalk has a healing quality about it. Now, take the chalk and draw a picture that symbolizes your anxiety... It doesn't matter what the picture is, whether it has a recognizable shape or whether it is shapeless and it makes no sense... The drawing simply needs to symbolize your anxiety, whatever that looks like... Everybody's' drawings will be different... Really spend some time on this drawing... You're doing a great job... (Allow yourself as much time as needed.)

When the picture is complete, sit back and look at it... While you look at it continue to breathe slowly and deeply, keeping your body very relaxed... Now, walk back to the chalkboard and pick up the eraser that is sitting in the chalk tray... Tell the anxiety you have drawn, "I am wiping you out of my life. You will no longer have a hold on me. Good-bye!" Then, see yourself erase the symbol on the chalkboard until it is completely gone. Great, you did it! Feel the release in your body as the symbol of anxiety on the chalkboard disappears.

VISUALIZATION ACTIVITY: CREATING INNER PEACE

Replace that space in your body where the anxiety was with a symbol of peace... See yourself walk back over to the chalkboard and pick up a piece of chalk... Again feel the healing source of the chalk as you hold it with your fingers... Now, create a symbol that encompasses inner peace... Again, everybody's pictures will look different... Spend some time drawing this image on the chalkboard... Feel a shower of peace come over your body as you stand back and look at the completed image of inner peace you drew on the chalkboard... Take as much time as you need to internalize and absorb this inner peace... Breathe it in... Feel the image come off the chalkboard and blanket your body... Be aware of the love and serenity that emanates from the image... Now allow the image to enter your body to fill up the space where the anxiety used to be... Just sit for a while with this new gift of inner peace, love, and serenity... Now, take a moment to again focus on your deep and relaxed breathing... When you feel comfortable, you may open your eyes. You will recall all the necessary details to complete this exercise. Whenever you feel anxious use this visualization exercise to bring yourself back to a peaceful place.

Write about this experience from beginning to end.

_____
_____
_____
_____
_____
_____
_____
_____
_____
_____
_____
_____
_____
_____
_____
_____
_____

Draw the symbol of your anxiety. After completing the drawing, shade over the picture as though you are erasing it.

Draw a picture of your symbol for inner peace. Take a moment to once again focus on it while you take in slow deep breaths.

To prevent slipping back into body-hatred and a negative body image, it is important to continue to practice and do the various activities and techniques we have shared with you to create healing.

THE LOVE YOUR BODY SUCCESS PLAN

Always remember you are a very special and unique creation of God, and you deserve peace, joy, happiness and a healthy life.

As an additional tool, we created the *Love Your Body Success Plan* as a helpful tool to refer to on a daily basis. Carefully read it over and fill in the blanks. Remember, the more you put into your own healing process, the more you will get out of it.

A. List ten affirmations that work well for you (5 body affirmations, 5 character affirmations). Commit to saying these to yourself in the mirror every day.

1._____
2._____
3._____
4._____
5._____

6._____

7._____

8._____

9._____

10._____

B. List 5 nurturing activities you enjoy. Commit to engaging in one activity on a daily basis. (It does not have to be the same activity every day; variety is good.) My nurturing activities are:

1._____

2._____

3._____

4._____

5._____

C. Depending upon your old relationship with food, either restricting or bingeing, will determine how you challenge yourself with food. For those of you who are restrictors write down three foods that you will challenge yourself to eat, without guilt and in moderation, over the next three weeks. If you are a binger, write down three binge foods that you will safeguard yourself against by not keeping them in your house during this vulnerable time of learning new and healthier behaviors.

1._____

2._____

3._____

D. Use the *"Thought-Stopping"* **technique (See Chapter 6) if you catch yourself engaging in negative self-talk.**

E. Be active in changing any negative thought to a positive thought. A positive frame of mind is a treasured gift to give yourself.

I, _____, commit to practice my above success plan for a minimum of 30 days.

At day 30 of working your *Love Your Body Success Plan*, document any changes you have experienced and retake *The Body Image Assessment* (at the end of this chapter) as a post-test.

_____

_____

_____

_____

_____

_____

_____

THE BODY IMAGE SUCCESS TRIANGLE

The *Body Image Success Triangle*, below, consists of three key elements: positive thinking, healthy eating, and self-nurturing. At the top of the triangle is positive thinking, since it is the basis for positive feelings and positive behaviors. By thinking positively, we cultivate positive expectations. With positive thinking, we are able to get through rough times because we know they are only temporary. When we think positive thoughts about our body, we treat it well. In contrast, negative thinking undermines our attempts at success. We question ourselves, become unsure, and can undo any progress we have made. Positive thinking does not come naturally for someone with a poor body image, but you can train yourself to think positively (See *"Thought-Stopping"* Chapter Six). By disciplining your thinking, you create an enormous opportunity for change.

Figure 9.5: Body Image Success Triangle

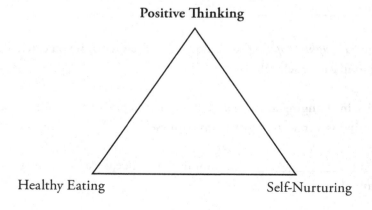

Positive Thinking

Healthy Eating   Self-Nurturing

Healthy eating, the second element of the *Body Image Success Triangle*, is a result of taking the time to take care of your body. When we listen to our body, we feed it healthy food on a regular basis. Healthy eating is linked to positive thinking, in that when we think positive thoughts we tend to engage in positive behaviors, such as feeding ourselves nourishing food. On the other hand, the better we eat the better we think and feel. Food affects mood. Healthy eating includes having a good relationship with food. This means we enjoy food and are not afraid to eat, and we don't worry that we will blow up with each bite.

Along with positive thinking and healthy eating is the third element: self-nurturing. A woman who loves and respects her body takes loving care of it by engaging in self-nurturing activities. She takes the time for fun, for playful, uplifting activities. Practicing self-nurturing regularly reinforces the message to your body that you love it and are treating it right. Success can be yours when you put into practice the elements of the *Body Image Success Triangle*.

Remember, the emphasis here is to LOVE yourself and your body. This requires engaging in loving behaviors and exercises. The next activity is for you to write yourself a love letter. We want you to really pour it on thick! In this letter, tell yourself all the terrific things about you and how special you are. You are a special gift to the world and are wonderful just the way you are. If you have some difficulty, try thinking about the wonderful things a good friend would say about you if they were asked to describe you. Make this the type of love letter you have always dreamed of receiving from that special someone. As you write the letter, imagine you are writing it to someone you really love, admire, and think is super special. Imagine the pleasure this person will get from reading this letter. Now, go back through your letter and remove any negativities or self-criticisms you may find. (Sometimes they mysteriously find their way in there.)

To love yourself and your body you must engage in loving behaviors and exercises.

LOVE LETTER TO ME

_____

_____

_____

_____

_____

_____

_____

_____

_____

_____

_____

_____

_____

_____

_____

_____

_____

_____

_____

_____

_____

_____

1. How do you feel after writing this letter?

_____

_____

_____

_____

_____

_____

_____

_____

Every day for one full week or more, read your love letter to yourself while looking into your eyes in the mirror. Use the *"Thought-Stopping"* technique, Chapter Six, if any negative thoughts surface during the exercise. Allow yourself to internalize the compliments and positive statements in your letter. Each day after reading your love letter, journal the thoughts and feelings you experienced while reading the love letter.

Day 1

_____

_____

Day 2

_____

_____

Day 3

_____

_____

Day 4

_____

_____

Day 5

_____

_____

Day 6

_____

_____

Day 7

_____

_____

Work your *Love Your Body Success Plan* for continued success. Give loving praise to your body and enjoy your new relationship with it.

It's time to re-evaluate your body image. Take *The Body Image Assessment,* as a post-test, (Figure 9.6). This is the same assessment you took at the beginning of the book. The assessment will give you a number you can compare with your original assessment to see if there has been a shift in your body image. Remember the lower the score, the better your body image is.

Figure 9.6: The Body Image Assessment

Instructions: For each of the following statements, rate the degree to which it applies to you. Circle only one number for each statement. After rating yourself on all statements, total your points to get your "Body Image" score.

#	Question	Never	Sometimes	Often	Always
Negative Thoughts/Feelings					
1	I feel ashamed of my body in the presence of a special person.	0	1	2	3
2	I feel that other people must think my body is ugly.	0	1	2	3
3	When I walk into a room, I feel the first thing people notice is my weight.	0	1	2	3
4	I feel that friends and family are embarrassed to be seen with me.	0	1	2	3
5	When I feel fat, I have a bad day.	0	1	2	3
	Subtotal				

#	Question	Never	Sometimes	Often	Always
Negative Self-Perception					
1	I don't like my body.	0	1	2	3
2	I avoid participating in sports or outside exercise because of my appearance.	0	1	2	3
3	I don't like looking at myself in the mirror.	0	1	2	3
4	I don't like to be looked at in public.	0	1	2	3

5	Enjoying activities is difficult because I am self-conscious about my appearance.	0	1	2	3
	Subtotal				

Destructive Behaviors/Patterns					
1	I compare my body to others to see if they are heavier than me.	0	1	2	3
2	Shopping for clothes makes me weight-focused and is therefore unpleasant.	0	1	2	3
3	I am preoccupied with feeling guilty about my weight.	0	1	2	3
4	The number on the scale determines how I feel about myself.	0	1	2	3
	Subtotal				
Now total the number of points you have circled in each column					
					Total Points

Appendix

❧

FOOD FOR THOUGHT

As this book comes to a close, we want to share some words of inspiration. Some participants of the *Love Your Body* Workshop have been gracious in allowing us to share some of their positive affirmations with you. Each individual granted permission for their affirmations to be printed in this book. Affirmations are powerful and can facilitate positive growth. As we mentioned before, the important thing to remember is that you need to be consistent with them. We would like to thank the workshop participants for sharing their affirmations.

Love Your Body Workshop Affirmations

I am wonderful just the way I am. (E. K. T.)

I am healthy and full. (D. W.)

I am beautiful. (J. R.)

I am worth more than I can imagine. (T. H.)

I am a unique child of God. (A. J.)

I am full of joy and happiness. (L. R. M.)

I am worthy and deserving of care and attention. (M. K. M.)

I accept and embrace myself. (E. K. T.)

My smile is infectious. (J. R.)

My body allows me to be mobile. (L. J.)

My body has its own strength and grace. (M. K. M.)

I have been blessed with many talents. (A. J.)

I admire my hands and fingers because they are long, graceful, sensitive and expressive. (E. K. T.)

I am a caring person and am loved by many. (A. J.)

My body is beautiful, and I will love and nurture it. (J. B.)

I am a loving person. (N. P.)

I treat myself with the respect I deserve. (L. R. M.)

I choose to look at the beauty life has to offer. (R. K.)

I have a gorgeous hour-glass figure. (P. N.)

I admire the curvature of my hips. (T. L.)

My hair is silky and resilient. (T. L.)

My smile accentuates the beauty of my face. (K. B.)

My arms flow through the air with elegance and grace. (S. B.)

My body is attractive to me. (S. B.)
I have cute toes. (F. K.)
I like the roundness of my tummy. (B. K.)
My thighs are a symbol of strength. (D. H.)
I choose to shower my body with positive messages. (E. M.)
I feel at one with my body. (T. L.)
I have pretty fingernails. (P. N.)
I have expressive and friendly eyes. (K. B.)
My freckles add character to my face. (F. K.)
I feel secure in my femininity. (B. K.)
My womanly figure is a gift from God. (T. L.)
I possess both beauty and strength. (J. B.)

Utilize some of these affirmations if you have difficulty getting started on your own. Writing affirmations to, and for, you is a little difficult at first; however, it becomes a lot easier with practice.

POEMS FOR REFLECTION

The following sections are inspirational writings and poems we wrote and wanted to share with you. These poems were written for the *Love Your Body* Workshop.

No Body's Perfect

This thought keeps running through my mind,
And yet it is so hard to find
A sense of love and inner peace with my body.
If "no body's perfect", why don't I embrace
My beautiful face?
Why don't I cherish my body and its space?
Lavish it in all its grace?
My body and spirit are me.
I can unite them and be free.
What I realized is
Loving my body is a choice; it's up to me.

Tami Brannon-Quan, Ph.D., C.A.S., M.F.T.

Who Am I?

Who am I?
Is this soft lullaby
I often hear.

What do I see
When I look at me?
I am a child of God.
I have a unique soul
And my Creator is in control.
He gave me special gifts
And is there to love me and uplift.

God gave me a body to house my spirit.
Why do I do the things I do to it?
My body loves me
And allows me to be free
To move about in our world.
My body and soul are unique creations
I will embrace them without hesitation.

Tami Brannon-Quan, Ph.D., C.A.S, M.F.T.

Creating My Own Smile

Hello, Sunshine!
I love you, you are divine.
Just look at that smile!
I can stare at it for awhile.

Your eyes twinkle and glisten
Because I know how to listen
To ME!

I hear your wants and needs
And I listen to your pleas
For you are now a priority.

This is what makes me happy.
It may sound kind of sappy,
But this I do to create my own smile
For now it lasts for a long, long while…

Tami Brannon-Quan, Ph.D., C.A.S., M.F.T.

No Time For Body Shame

I love my body!
Does that sound strange?
No time for negatives,
No time to rearrange.

It gets me where I'm going
Here and there throughout the day.
I'm grateful for my body,
No matter what they say.

Some treat their body with contempt;

All that hating is sure weird.
They struggle to control it
Like it's something to be feared.

But my hope for all of us
Is to be rid of grief and blame.
To live our lives freely
Without the body shame.

Lisa Licavoli, R.D., C.C.N.

PRAYER FOR MY BODY

Dear God,

I need your help! You have given me the gift of life, you have given me my body. What a generous gift. With this gift I can do all kinds of things. I can jump and swim and run and skip. I can eat and sleep and work and play. I can travel all over the world if I want with this body of mine.

Yet, why am I so unkind to it? Why do I criticize it and call it names? Why do I do things to hurt it and let others hurt it, too? This is no way to treat your precious gift.

From this moment forward, with your help, I will do everything in my power to cherish, honor, respect, and love my body. I will feed it nourishing foods, get plenty of rest, play more, and speak highly of it. I will treat it as the gift it is.

Amen

Lisa Licavoli, R.D., C.C.N.

NATIONAL NON-PROFIT EATING DISORDER ORGANIZATIONS

ANAD (National Association of Anorexia Nervosa and Associated Disorders)
PO Box 7
Highland Park, IL 60035
(847) 831-3438
www.anad.org
Distributes listings of therapists, hospitals and information materials; sponsors support groups, conferences, advocacy campaigns, research and crisis hotline.

ANRED (Anorexia Nervosa and Related Eating Disorders)
www.anred.com
Provides basic information, workshops, individual and professional training, community education, and a monthly newsletter.

Eating Disorder Referral and Information Center
2923 Sandy Point #6
Del Mar, CA 92014
(858) 792-7463
www.edreferral.com
Provides treatment referrals and information for all forms of eating disorders. A valuable resource!

EDA (Eating Disorders Anonymous)
18233 N. 16th Way
Phoenix, AZ 85022
www.eatingdisordersanonymous.org
A "balance, not abstinence" 12-step fellowship. Free literature available.

IAEDP (International Association of Eating Disorders Professionals)
P.O. Box 1295
Pekin, IL 61555-1295
(800) 800-8126
www.iaedp.com
A non-profit membership organization for professionals; provides certification,

education, local chapters, a newsletter and an annual conference.

www.HealthyBodyImage.com

The mission is to help people learn to nurture their body, mind and spirit in order to attain optimum health and fitness. Services provided include: individual psychotherapy, nutrition counseling, and The *Love Your Body* Workshop.

NEDA (National Eating Disorders Association)

603 Stewart St., Suite 803
Seattle, WA 98101
(800) 931-2237
www.nationaleatingdisorders.org

OA (Overeaters Anonymous Headquarters)

World Services Office
PO Box 44020
Rio Rancho, NM 87174-4020
(505) 891-2664
www.oa.org
A 12 step, self-help fellowship; free local meetings are listed in the white pages telephone book under "Overeaters Anonymous."

Bibliography

Beck, A. T. (1976). Cognitive Therapy and the Emotional Disorders. New York, N.Y.: International University Press.

Brannon-Quan, T. & Licavoli, L. (1996). Love Your Body Workshop: Facilitator handbook. Newport Beach, CA.: Esteem Publishing.

Brannon-Quan, T. & Licavoli, L. (1996). Love Your Body Workshop: Participant workbook. Newport Beach, CA.: Esteem Publishing.

Bruch, H. (1981). Development Considerations of Anorexia Nervosa and Obesity. Canadian Journal of Psychiatry, 26, 212-216.

Burns, D. D. (1993). Ten Days to Self-Esteem. New York, N.Y.: Quill William Morrow.

Cash, T. F. & Pruzinsky, T. (1990). Body Images: Development deviance and change. New York, NY.: The Guilford Press.

Cash, T. F. (1995). What Do You See When You Look in the Mirror?: Helping yourself to a positive body image. New York, NY: Bantam Books.

Clark, C. N. (1996). Food Fight: Calling a truce with disordered eating. The Physician and Sports Medicine, 24, 13-14.

Cooke, K. (1996). Real Gorgeous: The truth about body and beauty. New York, NY: W.W. Norton & Company, Inc.

David, M. (1991). Nourishing Wisdom: A mind-body approach to nutrition and well being. New York, NY.: Bell Tower.

Day, D. (1990). Young Women in Nova Scotia: A study of attitudes, behavior and aspirations. Halifax: Nova Scotia Advisory Counsel on the Status of Women.

Dixon, M. (1994). Love the Body You Were Born With: A ten-step workbook for women. New York, NY.: A Perigee Book.

Freedman, R. (1988). Bodylove: Learning to like our looks and ourselves. New York, NY.: Perennial Library.

Garner, D. M. & Garfinkel, P. E. (1985). Handbook of Psychotherapy for Anorexia Nervosa and Bulimia. New York, NY.: The Guilford Press.

Hall, L. (1993). Full Lives: Women who have freed themselves from food and weight obsession. Carlsbad, CA: Gurze Books.

Hutchinson, M. G. (1985). Transforming Body Image: Learning to love the body you have. Freedom, CA.: The Crossing Press.

Jasper, K. (1993). Monitoring and Responding to Media Messages. Eating Disorders: The Journal of Treatment and Prevention, 1, 109-114.

Keys, A., Brozek, J., Henschel, A., Mickelsen, O., & Taylor, H. L. (1950). The Biology of Human Starvation. Minneapolis: University of Minnesota Press.

Licavoli, L. (1995). Dietetics Goes into Therapy: Nutrition therapists replace rules with understanding. Journal of the American Dietetic Association, 95, 751-752.

Louden, J. (1992). The Woman's Comfort Book: A self-nurturing guide for restoring balance in your life. San Francisco, CA.: Harper, San Francisco.

McFarland, B. & Baker-Baumann, T. (1990). Shame and Body Image: Culture and the compulsive eater. Deerfield Beach, FL.: Health Communications, Inc.

Mellin, L., McNutt, S., Hu, Y., Schreiber, G. B., Crawford, P., & Obarzanek, E. (1991). A longitudinal study of dietary practices of black and white girls 9 and 10 years old at enrollment: The NHLBI growth and health study. Journal of Adolescent Health, 27-37.

Mellin, L., Scully, S., & Irwin, C. (1986). Disordered Eating Characteristics in Pre-adolescent Girls. Paper presented at the American Dietetic Association Meeting.

Murray, S. H., Touyz, S. W., & Beumont, P. J. V. (1996). Awareness and Perceived Influence of Body Ideals in the Media: A comparison of eating disorder patients and the general community. Eating Disorders: The Journal of Treatment and Prevention, 4, 33-46.

Newman, L. (1991). Some Body to Love: A guide to loving the body you have. Chicago, IL.: Third Side Press.

Newmark, G. R. (1994). Healing Body Image with Yoga. Yoga Journal, 114, 17-19, 114.

Patton, G. C. (1992). Eating Disorders: Antecedents, evolution, and course. Annals of Medicine, 24, 281-285.

Peters, P., Amos, R., Hoerr, S., Koszewski, W., Huang, Y. & Betts, N. (1996). Questionable Dieting Behaviors Are Used by Young Adults Regardless of Sex or Student Status. Journal of American Dietetic Association, 96, 709-711.

Polivy, J. & Herman, C. P. (1985). Dieting and Bingeing: A causal analysis. American Psychologist, 40, 193-201.

Rodin, J., Silberstein, L., & Streigel-Moore, R. (1984). Women and Weight: A normative discontent. Nebraska Symposium on Motivation, 32, 267-307.

Shisslak, C. M., Crago, M., & Estes, L. S. (1995). The spectrum of eating disturbances. International Journal of Eating Disorders, 18 (3), 209-219.

Smith, A. (1996). The Female Athlete Triad: Causes, diagnosis, and treatment. The Physician and Sports Medicine, 24, 67-86.

Smolak, L. (1996). National Eating Disorders Association/Next Door Neighbors puppet guide book.

Stake, J., & Lauer, M. L. (1987). The Consequences of Being Overweight: A controlled study of gender differences. Sex Roles, 16, 435-446.

Tribole, E. & Resch, E. (1995). Intuitive Eating: A recovery book for the chronic dieter. New York, NY.: St. Martin's Press.

Vandereycken, W. (1993). The Sociocultural Roots of the Fight Against Fatness: Implications for eating disorders and obesity. Eating Disorders: The Journal of Treatment and Prevention, 1, 7-16.

Williamson, D. A. (1990). Assessment of Eating Disorders: Obesity, anorexia and bulimia nervosa. New York, NY.: Pergamon Press.

Wolf, N. (1991). The Beauty Myth: How images of beauty are used against women. New York, NY.: Anchor Books.

Printed in the United States
by Baker & Taylor Publisher Services